QUICK REVIEW OF BIOMECHANICS

(For Under Graduate Physiotherapy Students)

First Edition

AJAY YADAV

M.P.T. (Musculoskeletal), M. Phil

Member Indian Society of Biomechanics

Member Indian Association of Physiotherapists

Printed by CreateSpace, An Amazon.com Company

Available from Amazon.com, CreateSpace.com, and other retail outlets

Copyright © 2015 AJAY YADAV

All rights reserved.

ISBN-13: 978-1511512121

ISBN-10: 1511512121

Dedicated to

``MAA KAMAKHYA``

My Family, Teachers

Friends, Students

&

Prajana, Aniketh

PREFACE

The book entitled `Quick Review of Biomechanics`, has flavor of its own both, in scope and content distinctly different from a number of already existing books in the market. The major thrust has been given to make the book more students friendly. Topics have been explained according to the syllabus avoiding unnecessary details. Any suggestions for further improvement of the book will be highly appreciated.

Ajay Yadav

ACKNOWLEDGEMENTS

I, first of all, express my gratitude and thank the people those worked hard with me to complete this project successfully in time. I don`t have the words to express my thanks to my family, friends and colleagues who initiated and motivated me to start this project. .

I express my special thanks to American Physical Therapy Association for giving permission to use some materials from their journal. And I also extend my thanks to management, colleague, students and well-wishers of Doon (PG) Paramedical College & Hospital, Dehradun, India who encouraged, helped and guided to create one venture in my life. And I also thanks to CreateSpace, an Amazon.com Company.

Thanks to all, I need your help too to continue my achievement.

CONTENTS

Basic Concepts of Biomechanics-------------------------------1

Biomechanics of Upper Limb-------------------------------21

Biomechanics of Lower Limb-------------------------------40

Biomechanics of Trunk--------------------------------------68

Biomechanics of Gait--74

Biomechanics of Posture-------------------------------------80

Biomechanics of Prosthetic----------------------------------85

BIOMECHANICAL CONCEPTS

Mechanics: Mechanics is the branch of science that deals with forces and effects of forces, specifically the motion and deformation of solid, liquid and gaseous.

Biomechanics: (Greek bio meaning way of life and mechanics)

"Biomechanics is a branch of science that deals with forces and the effect of forces on living system and matter."

Biomechanics has been defined as the study of the movement of living things using the science of mechanics (Hatze, 1974).

Biomechanics represents an amalgamation of several different fields including mechanics, physics, engineering, anatomy, physiology, and mathematics.

KINEMATICS**

Kinematics: Kinematics is the area of biomechanics that includes descriptions of motion without regard for the forces producing the motion. **[It studies only the movements of the body.]**

Kinematics variables for a given movement may include following:

1. Type of motion.
2. Location of motion.
3. Direction of motion.
4. Magnitude of motion.
5. Rate or Duration of motion.

Mass

Mass is a property of a physical body which determines the strength of its mutual gravitational attraction to other bodies, its resistance to being accelerated by a force, and in the theory of relativity gives the mass–energy content of a system. The SI unit of mass is the kilogram (kg).

Rigid Body

A collection of particles occupying fixed locations with respect to each other. The assumption is that a rigid body will not deform under the action of an applied force however large the force may be. Obviously, this is an approximation in every case because all known materials deform by some amount under the action of a force.

Center of Mass

The point on a body that moves in the same way that a particle subject to the same external forces would move.

Centre of Gravity (COG)

The **COG** is a hypothetical point at which all mass would appear to be concentrated and is the point at which the force of gravity would appear to act.

In a symmetrical object, the COG is located in the geometric center of the object. In an asymmetrical object, the COG will be located toward the heavier end where the mass will be evenly distributed around the point.

Line of Gravity (LOG)

The action line and direction of the force of gravity on an object are always vertically downward toward the center of the earth regardless of the orientation in space of the object. The gravity vector is commonly referred to as the line of gravity (LOG). The LOG is an imaginary vertical line through the center of gravity.

Base of Support (BOS)

The base of support (BOS), as applied to a rigid body, is the area by which it is supported.

For an object to be stable, the LOG must fall within the BOS. When the LOG falls outside the BOS, the object will fall. When the BOS of an object is large, the LOG has more freedom to move without passing beyond the limits of the base.

- ✓ The larger the BOS of an object, the greater the stability of that object.
- ✓ The closer the COG of the object is to the BOS, the more stable is the object.
- ✓ An object cannot be stable unless its LOG falls within its BOS.

Moment of Inertia

The rotational equivalent of mass in its mechanical effect, that is, the resistance to a change of state (a speeding up or slowing down) during rotation. Intuitively, this would appear to be dependent on the mass of the object and the way the mass is distributed. In fact, the effect of distribution of mass is dominant as the following formula indicates:

$$I = m \cdot r^2$$

Where m = mass and r = distance from axis of rotation.

Linear Motion

In which all parts of the body travel along parallel paths. This does not imply motion in a straight line that is known as rectilinear translation. Linear motion along a curved path (curvilinear translation) is possible as long as the body does not rotate.

Angular Motion

Motion that is not linear. If the axis of rotation is fixed, all particles in the body travel in a circular manner. If the axis of rotation is not fixed, the motion is actually a combination of translation and rotation.

Scalar

A quantity that only has magnitude. For example, mass, length, or kinetic energy are scalar quantities and can be manipulated with conventional arithmetic.

Vector

A quantity that has both direction and magnitude.

A force, for example, is always described by how big it is and by the direction in which it is acting. Velocity is also a vector quantity because it expresses the rate of change of position in a given direction.

Displacement

The change in the position of a body. This change may be translations, whereby every point of the body is displaced along parallel lines; it may be rotational, with the points of the body describing concentric circles around an axis; or it may be a combination of the two.

Velocity

A measure of a body's motion in a given direction. Because velocity has both magnitude and direction, it is a vector quantity that can be positive, negative, or zero. Linear velocity is the rate at which a body moves in a straight line.

Angular Velocity

The rate of movement in rotation calculated as the first time derivative of angular displacement.

Acceleration

The rate of change of velocity with respect to time, mathematically the second time derivative of displacement and the first time derivative of velocity. Acceleration is also a vector quantity that may take positive, negative, or zero values.

Angular Acceleration

Angular acceleration refers to the rate at which the angular velocity of a body changes with respect to time. In algebraic form, average angular acceleration is equal to the final angular velocity minus the initial angular velocity divided by the time taken.

Force[**]

Force:

Force is a push or pull exerted by one material object or substance on another.

Force is that which alters the state of rest of a body or its uniform motion in a straight line.

External forces are pushes or pulls on the body that arises from sources outside the body.

Gravity is an external force that under normal conditions constantly affects all objects.

Internal forces are forces that act on the body but arise from sources within the human body. Examples are muscles, ligaments, and bones. Internal forces are essential to human function because external forces are difficult to depend on to create purposeful movement of a body segment. Internal forces serve to counteract those external forces that jeopardize the integrity of human joint structure.

Resultant Force

The **resultant force** is the difference between the two forces acting in opposite directions on an object. The **resultant force** is zero if both forces are equal.

Equilibrium

That condition when the resultant force and moment acting on a body are zero.

Moment Arm

The perpendicular distance from the point of application of a force to the axis of rotation.

Moment

The turning effect produced by a force. Calculated as the product of the force and the perpendicular distance between the point of application of the force and the axis of rotation. In vector terms, the calculation is the vector (cross) product of force and distance.

Couple

An arrangement of two equal and opposite parallel forces that tend to cause rotation. When a couple is exerted on a body, it tends to produce angular acceleration. The magnitude of the turning moment is equal to the product of the size of the forces and the perpendicular distance between their lines of action. This distance between the lines of action of the two forces is called the **moment arm.**

Levers of the Human Body

A lever is a rigid bar, which is capable of movement about a fixed point called a **Fulcrum** (F). Work is done when a force or effort (E), applied at one point on the lever, acts upon another force or weight (W), acting at a second point on the lever. The perpendicular distance from the fulcrum to the effort (E) may be called the **effort's arm** and that from the fulcrum to the weight (W) as the weight's arm.

In the body a lever is represented by a bone, which is capable of movement about a fulcrum formed at the articulating surfaces of a joint; the effort which works the lever is supplied by the force of muscle contraction, applied at the point of insertion to the bone, while the weight may be either at the centre of gravity of the part moved, or of the object to be lifted.

There are three Orders or Classes of levers, each of which is characterized by the relative positions of the fulcrum, effort, and weight.

First – Class Levers:

The fulcrum is between the effort and the weight; it may be situated centrally, or towards either the effort or weight. The feature of this Order is **stability**, and a state of equilibrium can be achieved either with or without mechanical advantage.

Examples:

1) During nodding movements of the head Lever – Skull, Fulcrum – Atlanto-occipital joint, Weight – Anteriorly in face, Effort – Contraction of posterior neck muscles

2) During tilting movements of pelvis, Lever – Pelvis, Fulcrum – Hip joint, Weight – Body weight, Effort – Contraction of hip extensor muscles

Second – Class Levers:

The weight is between the fulcrum and the effort, and the effort's arm must therefore always exceed the weight's arm. This is the **lever of power** as there must always be mechanical advantage.

Examples :-

1. When heels are raised to stand on toes, Lever – Tarsals and metatarsals, Fulcrum – Metatarophalangeal joint, Weight – Body weight is transmitted through ankle joint to talus, Effort – At insertion of tendo-calcaneum by contraction of calf muscles
2. During action of brachioradialis muscle in flexing the elbow joint, Lever – Humerus, Fulcrum – Elbow joint, Weight – Situated in forearm bones Effort – At insertion of tendon of brachioradialis by its contraction

Third – Class Levers:

The effort is between the fulcrum and the weight, and the weight's arm must therefore exceed the effort's arm. This type of lever, in which there is always a mechanical disadvantage, is **the lever of velocity**.

E g:-

1) When Lever – Forearm, Fulcrum – Elbow joint Weight – Some object held in hand Effort – Contraction of brachialis muscle applied at its insertion it can be seen that small amount of muscular contraction will be translated into much more extensive and rapid movement at hand.

2) When Lever – Leg, Fulcrum – Knee joint Weight – Some weight applied at the foot Effort – Contraction of hamstring muscles applied at its insertion it can be seen that small amount of muscular contraction will be translated into much more extensive and rapid movement of the foot.

Mechanical Advantage

The mechanical advantage of a lever is the ratio of the length of the lever on the applied force side of the fulcrum to the length of the lever on the resistance force side of the fulcrum. There are three types of levers- class 1, class 2, and class 3.

How to calculate the Mechanical Advantage in a Lever

1. Identify the fulcrum. This will be the point about which the the board or rigid object pivots around.
2. Identify the locations of the input and output forces. The input force is the force that is applied to the lever, oftentimes by a machine or human. The output force is the force that the lever exerts onto an object.
3. Find the distance between the fulcrum and the input force. This is known as the resistance arm.
4. Find the distance from the fulcrum to the output force. This is known as the effort arm.
5. Divide the length of the effort arm by the length of the resistance arm to calculate mechanical advantage.

    MA = L (effort arm) / L(resistance arm)

A ratio of 1 indicates no change in mechanical advantage, less than 1 a decrease, and greater than 1 an increase in mechanical advantage. A first-class lever can therefore have any value for mechanical advantage, a second-class lever always has a value greater than 1, and a third class lever always has a value less than 1.

Only class 1 or class 2 levers can be used to gain a mechanical advantage.

Weight

The force that results from the action of a gravitational field on a mass. Weight can be thought of as the force an object exerts on a stationary supporting surface placed perpendicular to a gravitational field (and by Newton's third law as the force the surface exerts on the object).

Friction

The tangential force acting between two bodies in contact that opposes motion or impending motion. If the two bodies are at rest, then the frictional forces are called **static friction**. If there is relative motion between the two bodies, then the forces acting between the surfaces are called **kinetic friction**. Two types of friction exist: dry friction, also called coulomb friction, and fluid friction.

Joint Forces

The forces that exist between the articular surfaces of the joint. Joint forces are the result of muscle forces, gravity, and inertial forces (usually, muscle forces are responsible for the largest part).

Reaction Forces

The equal and opposite forces that exist between adjacent bones at a joint caused by the weight and inertial forces of the two segments. Joint reaction force is a fairly abstract concept useful in mathematical analysis but not much use in practice. This quantity must not be confused with joint forces that include the effects of muscle action.

Ground Reaction Forces

The forces that act on the body as a result of interaction with the ground. Newton's third law implies that ground reaction forces are equal and opposite to those that the body is applying to the ground. Ground reaction forces can be measured with a force platform.

Inertial Forces

The product of the mass of a body and its acceleration or the moment of inertia and the angular acceleration.

Gravitational Force

The force exerted on an object as a result of gravitational pull. This force may be considered as a single force representing the sum of all the individual weights within the object.

Center of Pressure

A quantity available from a force platform describing the centroid of the pressure distribution. It can be thought of as (and is sometimes called) the point of application of the force, but this is a somewhat misleading definition unless the force is truly applied at a point (eg, by the tip of a walking cane). In the more general case, the force is applied over a diffuse area (eg, the plantar aspect of the foot).

KINETICS**

Kinetics: Kinetics is the area of biomechanics concerned with the forces producing motion or maintaining equilibrium. [**It studies the movements along with the forces, which produces the particular movement.**]

Newton's Laws

Three laws that form the basis of conventional or Newtonian Mechanics.

The laws can be remembered by the acronym **IN-MO-RE**:

1) First law of **IN**ertia,

2) Second law of **M**omentum

3) Third law of **RE**action.

Newton's first law states that a body will maintain a state of rest or uniform motion unless acted on by a net force.

Newton's second law states that the change in momentum of the body under the action of a resultant force will be proportional to the product of the magnitude of the force and the time for which it acts (i.e., the impulse). The second law also states that the change in momentum will be in the direction of the resultant force.

Newton's third law states that action and reaction are equal and opposite.

Impulse

The effect of a force acting over a period of time. Impulse is determined mathematically by the integral of the force-time curve, more simply thought of as the area under the force-time curve. Newton's second law allows us to quantify the effect of a force on the velocity of an object if we know the impulse by the impulse momentum relationship.

Linear Momentum

The product of the mass of an object and its linear velocity.

Angular Momentum

The rotational equivalent of linear momentum that can be thought of as describing the "amount of motion" that the body possesses during rotation.

Impulse-Momentum Relationship

The change in momentum experienced by a body under the action of a force is equal to the impulse of the resultant force. This follows directly from the definition of Newton's second law.

Work

Work is done when a force moves an object through a distance. Whenever a constant force exists and motion takes place in a straight line, then work equals the magnitude of the force (F) times the distance (d) through which the object moves: $W = F \cdot d$.

Power

The rate of doing work. Power is equal to the work done divided by the time during which the work is being done: $P = W/t$.

Energy

The capacity for doing work. In any system, this capacity cannot be destroyed, but energy can be transformed from one form to another (this is a statement of the Principle of Conservation of Energy). In biomechanics, the forms of energy that are most frequently encountered are kinetic energy, potential energy, strain energy, and heat energy.

Kinetic Energy

That component of the mechanical energy of a body resulting from its motion.

Potential Energy

That component of the mechanical energy of a body resulting from its position.

Potential Energy = m.g.h, where m is mass, g is acceleration resulting from gravity, and h is distance above datum.

Work—Energy Principle

The work done on a body is equal to the change in kinetic energy of the body. A more comprehensive statement is that the work done on the body is equal to the change in the energy level of the body.

Energy Level

The total mechanical energy of a body or system. This total represents the sum of the translational and rotational kinetic energy and the potential energy.

Energy level = KET + KER + PE

BIOMECHANICS OF TISSUES

Ligament

Ligaments are connective tissue structures that connect or bind one bone to another either at or near a joint.

- Ligaments are usually named descriptively according to their Location, Shape, Bony attachments and relationship to one another.
- Composed of a small amount of cells (about 20%), and a large extracellular matrix (about 80% to 90%).

Tendon:

Tendons connect muscle to bone. Tendons are composed of a small cellular component (primarily fibroblasts) and a large extracellular matrix.

Groups of fiber bundles enclosed by a loose connective tissue sheath are called the **Endotenon**.

The sheath that covers all secondary bundles or fascicles is called the **epitenon**..

The **peritenon** or **paratenon** is a double-layered sheath of areolar tissue that is loosely attached to the outer surface of the epitenon.

The peritenon may become a synovial-filled sheath called the **Tenosynovium** (or tendon sheath) in tendons located in the wrist and hand that are subjected to high levels of friction.

Cartilage

Cartilage is a connective tissue composed of cells (chondrocytes) and fibres (collagen or yellow elastic) embedded in firm, gel-like matrix, which is rich in a mucopolysacchrides.

Cartilage is usually divided into the following types:

1. White fibrocartilage
2. Yellow elastic cartilage
3. Hyaline articular cartilage

Bone

Bone is the hardest of all connective tissue found in the body.

It consists of a cellular component and an extracellular matrix consisting of an inter fibrillar component and a fibrillar component.

The cellular component consists of fibroblasts, fibrocytes, osteoblasts, osteocytes, osteoclasts, and osteoprogenitor cells.

The fibroblasts and fibrocytes are essential for the production of collagen.

The **osteoblasts** are primary bone forming cells that are responsible not only for synthesis of bone but also for its deposition and mineralization.

Osteoclasts are responsible for bone resorption.

General Properties of Connective Tissue

Viscoelasticity

Although connective tissue appears in many forms throughout the body, all connective tissue exhibits the common property of viscoelasticity. The behavior of viscoelastic materials is a combination of the properties of elasticity and viscosity.

Elasticity refers to a material's ability to return to its original state following deformation after removal of the deforming load.

The term elasticity implies that length changes or deformations are directly proportional to the applied forces or loads.

Viscosity refers to a material's ability to dampen shearing forces.

When forces are applied to viscous materials, the tissues exhibit time-dependent and rate-dependent properties.

Time-Dependent Properties:

When a viscoelastic material is subjected to either a constant compressive or tensile load, the material initially responds by rapidly deforming and then continues to deform over a finite length of time even if the load remains constant. Deformation of the tissue continues until a state of equilibrium is reached when the load is balanced. This phenomenon is called **creep effect**.

[Property of the human elastic structures to get deformed or reformed due to continuous prolonged stress is known as creep effect.]

Rate-Dependent Properties:

When a force is applied and then removed, some of the energy created during the stretching or compression of the material may be lost in the form of heat and therefore the material may not return to its original dimensions. The loss of energy (difference between energy expended and energy regained) is called hysteresis.

Viscoelastic materials exhibit hysteresis when they are subjected to the application and removal of forces.

Stress & Strain:

When loads (forces) are applied to a structure or material, forces are created within the structure or material that are called **mechanical stresses**.

Joints

Joint is a junction between two or more bones or cartilages.

It is a device to permit movements. The two broad categories of joints or arthroses are synarthroses (nonsynovial joints) and diarthroses (synovial joints).

Closed Kinematic Chain and Open Kinematic Chain

The system of joints and links is constructed so that motion of one link at one joint will produce motion at all of the other joints in the system in a predictable manner. This is known as **closed kinematic chain**. When the ends of the limbs or parts of the body are free to move without causing motion at another joint, the system is referred to as an **open kinematic chain**.

Arthrokinematic

The term **arthrokinematics** is used to refer to movements of joint surfaces. The terms roll, slide, and spin are used to describe the type of motion that the moving part performs. A **roll** refers to the rolling of one joint surface on another.

In the knee, the femoral condyles roll on the fixed tibial surface. **Sliding**, which is a pure translatory motion, refers to the gliding of one component over another. In the hand, the proximal phalanx slides over the fixed end of the metacarpal. The term **spin** refers to a rotation of the movable component. At the elbow, the head of the radius spins on the capitulum of the humerus during supination and pronation of the forearm.

Concavo-convex Rule: When a convex articulating surface moves on a stable concave surface, the sliding of the convex articulating surface occurs in the opposite direction to the motion of the bony lever. When a concave articulating surface is moving on a stable convex surface, sliding occurs in the same direction as motion of the bony lever.

[Convex surface = male articulating surface Concave surface = female articulating surface. If proximal part (bone) is moving and distal part is fixed, then movement of articular surfaces takes place in opposite direction to that of bony lever. Male articulating surface female articulating surface proximal distal moving stable movement of articular surface in opposite direction .If proximal part (bone) is stable and distal part is moving, then movement of articular surface takes place in the same direction to that of bony lever male articulating surface female articulating surface proximal distal stable moving movement of articular surface in same direction]

Instantaneous Axis of Rotation

The axis of rotation at any particular point in the motion is called the **instantaneous axis of rotation** (IAR) . IARs occur most notably when opposing articular surfaces are of unequal size.

Closed-Packed Position and Loose-Packed Position

All synovial joints have a closed-packed position in which the joint surfaces are maximally congruent and the ligaments and capsule are maximally taut. The **closed-packed position** is usually at the extreme end of a ROM. In the closed-packed position a joint possesses its greatest stability and is resistant to tensile forces that tend to cause distraction of the joint surfaces.

In the **loose-packed position** of a joint, the articular surfaces are relatively free to move in relation to one another. The loose-packed position of a joint is any position other than the closed-packed position, although the term is commonly used to refer to the position at which the joint structures are more lax and the joint cavity has a greater volume than in other positions.

Osteokinematics:

Osteokinematics refers to the movement of the bones rather than the movement of the articular surfaces. The normal ROM of a joint is sometimes called the anatomic or physiologic ROM , because it refers to the amount of motion available to a joint within the anatomic limits of the joint structure.

The extent of the anatomic range is determined by a number of factors, including the shape of the joint surfaces, the joint capsule, ligaments, muscle bulk, and surrounding musculotendinous and bony structures.

Hypermobility

It may be caused by a failure to limit motion by either the bony or soft tissues or results in instability.

Hypomobility

It may be caused by bony or cartilaginous blocks to motion or by the inability of the capsule, ligaments, or muscles to elongate sufficiently to allow a normal ROM.

A contracture, which is a term used to describe the shortening of soft tissue structures around a joint, is one cause of hypomobility.

MUSCLE MECHANICS**

Contraction

In muscles, an active shortening of the muscle resulting in a reduction in the distance between the two ends of a muscle. It has, however, become popular to use the term to imply development of tension by a muscle whether or not shortening is underway. This usage is inexact and is not encouraged.

Muscle Action

The development of muscle tension (more appropriate than the term "contraction"). It can be applied to any type of tension development regardless of whether a muscle is lengthening, shortening, or maintaining the same length.

Concentric Muscle Action

Muscle shortening under tension. This shortening occurs when the net moment developed by a muscle and its synergists is greater than the moment caused by the external forces acting on the segment to which the muscle is attached.

Isotonic Muscle Action

Muscle action that involves the production of a constant force. For in vivo muscle actions, the term is also commonly used both when the joint moment is constant over a range of motion and when a constant load is being moved through a distance. It is important to realize, however, that because of the leverage effects at the joint, the force developed by the muscles in both these cases will actually be changing, rendering them nonisotonic.

Isometric Muscle Action

Muscle action that involves no change in length of the muscle. This condition probably does not exist because the contractile components of a muscle shorten at the expense of the elastic structures in series even when the joint crossed by the muscle is fixed. The definition, therefore, is usually relaxed to mean the action of a muscle when no change exists in the distance between its points of attachment referring to the joint and not to the muscle.

Isokinetic Muscle Action

Muscle action in which the rate of shortening or lengthening of the muscle is constant. Because joint geometry makes this impossible to determine in vivo, the definition is usually relaxed to apply either to a constant velocity of the load being lifted or resisted or to a constant angular velocity of the joint.

Origin

The source or beginning of a muscle. The term generally refers to the more fixed end or the more proximal end.

Insertion

The more distal attachment of the muscle or the attachment that is more mobile. Again, this is an ambiguous term for which attachment should be substituted.

Muscular Efficiency

Expresses the ratio of the mechanical work done to the metabolic energy expended (a widely used term in biomechanics and physiology). This definition has many problems, most of which are related to the definition of the work done. The major stumbling blocks to the establishment of a relationship are the storage of elastic energy in muscles, the different metabolic costs of positive and negative work, and the energy transfer between body segments.

Spurt and Shunt Muscles

A muscle's ability to exert rotatory force on a limb. This classification has, however, been challenged. When the distal attachment is close to the joint at which the muscle acts, the muscle is called a spurt muscle. This is said to result in a greater rotatory component compared with its stabilizing component. The shunt muscles have their more proximal attachment close to the joint, and their action is said to be more for stabilization than for rotation. The biceps brachii muscle is often presented as an example of a spurt muscle and the brachioradialis muscle as an example of a shunt muscle.

Tension-Length Relationship

The cross-bridges can only form where thin and thick filaments already overlap, so that the **length** of the sarcomere has a direct influence on the force generated when the sarcomere shortens. This is also called the **length-tension relationship**.

MECHANICS OF MATERIALS**

Density

The mass of matter in a given space, that is, the mass per unit volume.

Note: Pure water at 0°C has a density of 1.0. Objects with a density greater than 1 will sink in water; those with a density less than 1 will float in water.

Tension

A loading mode in which collinear forces acting in opposite directions tend to pull an object apart. In general, a tensile force will cause the length of the body to be increased and the width to be narrowed.

Distraction

The movement of two surfaces away from each other. In joints, distraction refers to a form of dislocation where the two joint surfaces are separated but retain their ligamentous integrity.

Compression

A loading mode in which collinear forces are acting in opposite directions to push the material together. Compression usually results in a shortening and widening of the material.

Stress

Force per unit area that develops within a structure in response to externally applied loads. The stress may be tensile or compressive depending on the mode of loading. The stress may also be normal (changing the length in a structure) or shear (changing the angle in a structure).

Strain

Deformation that occurs at a point in a structure under loading. Two basic types of strain exist: normal strain, which is a change in length, and shear strain, which is a change in angle. Normal strain is the ratio of deformation (lengthening or shortening) to original length. Shear strain is the amount of angular deformation that occurs in a structure.

Modulus of Elasticity (Young's modulus)

The ratio of stress to strain at any point in the elastic region of deformation, yielding a value for stiffness. The stiffer the material, the higher the modulus. The moduli in compression and tension are different for most biological materials because they are anisotropic.

Elastic Deformation

A strain in a material that is entirely reversible when the stress is released.

Plastic Deformation

A strain in a material that is permanent and will not recover when the stress is released.

Strain Rate

The speed at which a strain-producing load is applied or the first derivative of strain.

Isotropic

A material that has no directional structure and exhibits the same mechanical properties when loaded in different directions. For example, in an isotropic material (eg, a sheet of natural rubber), the elastic properties are identical in all directions.

Anisotropic

A material that has a directional structure and exhibits different mechanical properties when loaded in different directions. For example, because the structure of bone or tendon is different in the transverse and the longitudinal directions, the modulus of elasticity varies according to the direction in which the load is imposed.

Bending

The result of applying a load to a structure such that it bends about an axis. The structure will be experiencing a combination of tension and compression on opposite surfaces.

Neutral Axis

The central plane in which the tensile and compressive stresses and strains resulting from bending equal zero.

Bending Moment

A quantitative measure of the tendency of a force to bend a structure.
It is calculated as the product of the applied force and the perpendicular distance from the point of force application to the axis.

Bone Remodeling

The ability of the bone to adapt, by changing its size, shape, and structure, to the mechanical demands placed on it. The idea that living bone can functionally adapt to internal stresses and strains was first advanced by Julius Wolff in 1884. Wolff's law states that bone is laid down where needed and resorbed where not needed. The remodeling may be either external (a change in the external shape of the bone) or internal (a change in the porosity, mineral content, and density of bone).

Fatigue

The failure of a material caused by loading.

Viscoelasticity

The behavior of materials that exhibit the features of hysteresis, stress relaxation, and creep.

Note: Modeling of viscoelastic behavior must include elements such as dashpots (fluid-filled damping units) that can absorb energy, whereas elastic behavior can be satisfactorily modeled by perfect springs, which return all the energy they store.

Hysteresis

A phenomenon in which a body, when subjected to cyclic loading, exhibits a stress-strain relationship during the loading process different from that in the unloading process.

Stress Relaxation

The phenomenon in which the stress in a sample, which was suddenly strained and then maintained at the final strain, gradually decreases with time.

Creep

Progressive deformation of soft tissues because of constant loading over an extended period of time. This is typically demonstrated by suddenly stressing a sample and then holding the load constant afterwards. If the sample continues to deform, then it is said to be exhibiting creep.

Shock Absorption

The progressive damping of an applied force. Damping is a complex, generally nonlinear, phenomenon that exists whenever energy is dissipated.

QUICK REVIEW OF BIOMECHANICS

MOVEMENTS

PLANES AND AXES OF MOTION

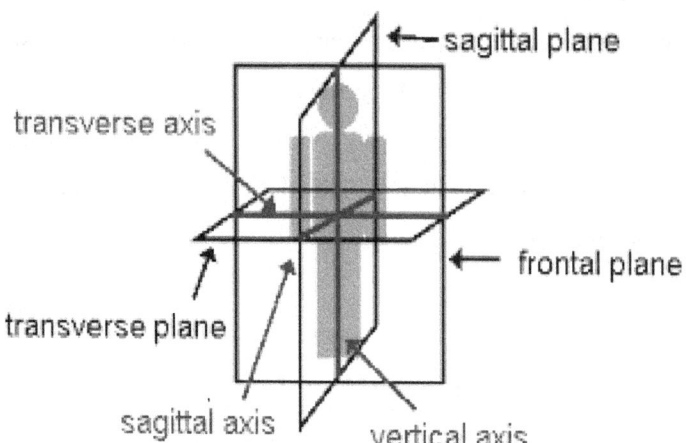

Depending on the joint, we must analyze the motion at just ONE, or TWO, but never more than THREE PLANES.

1. Sagittal
2. Frontal (sometimes called the coronal plane)
3. Transverse (sometimes called the horizontal plane)

Each plane is defined by an axis, a line that is perpendicular to the plane. When we observe a drawing of the joint in a single plane, we appreciate the joint's axis as a point; in the drawings linked above, an 'x' marks the joint axis.

PLANE	AXIS	MOVEMENT	SPECIAL CASES
Sagittal	Lateral*	Flexion Extension	Hyperextension Dorsiflexion/Plantar flexion of ankle
Frontal	A-P	Abduction Adduction	fingers/toes ulnar and radial deviation of wrist
Transverse	Vertical longitudinal	Rotation	Horizontal abduction of shoulder or hip
Multi-planar	Oblique	Pronation Supination	Subtalar joint Midtarsal joint Radio-ulnar joint

JOINT STRUCTURE

Three major types of joints in the body

1. FIBROUS JOINTS (SYNARTHROSES)
2. CARTILAGINOUS JOINTS (AMPHIARTHROSES)
3. SYNOVIAL JOINTS (DIARTHROSES)

Classification of joints

I. FIBROUS JOINTS (SYNARTHROSES)
   1. Sutures
   2. Syndesmoses
   3. Gomphoses
II. CARTILAGINOUS JOINTS (AMPHIARTHROSES)
   1. Synchondroses (Hyaline cartilage)
   2. Symphyses (Fibrocartilage)
III. SYNOVIAL JOINTS (DIARTHROSES)
   1. UNIAXIAL
      - Ginglymus (Hinge)
      - Trochoid (Pivot)
   2. BIAXIAL
      - Condyloid
      - Saddle
   3. TRIAXIAL
      - Ball and socket
      - Planar

References:

1. **Adapted from *Phys Ther*. 1984;64:1886-1902,with permission of the American Physical Therapy Association,© 1984 American Physical Therapy Association.
2. P. Levangie, C. Norkin,2000, *Joint Structure and Function: A Comprehensive Analysis*, F.A. Davis Company.
3. Hatze, Herbert (1974). "The meaning of the term biomechanics". *Journal of Biomechanics* 7: 189–190.
4. Martin, R. Bruce (October 23, 1999). "A genealogy of biomechanics". Presidential Lecture presented at the 23rd Annual Conference of the American Society of Biomechanics University of Pittsburgh, Pittsburgh PA. Retrieved 2 January 2014
5. Basmajian, J.V, & DeLuca, C.J. (1985) *Muscles Alive: Their Functions Revealed, Fifth edition*. Williams & Wilkins Publ.
6. *Doriand's Illustrated Medical Dictionary*, ed 25. Philadelphia, PA, WB Saunders Co, 1974
7. Frost HM: An Introduction to Biomechanics. Springfield, IL, Charles C Thomas, Publisher, 1967
8. Fung YC: *Biomechanics*: Mechanical Properties of Living Tissues. New York,NY, Springer-Verlag New York Inc, 1981
9. *Taber's Cyclopedic Medical Dictionary*, ed 11. Philadelphia, PA, FA Davis Co,1970
10. Frankel VH, Nordin M (eds): *Basic Biomechanics of the Skeletal System*.Philadelphia, PA, Lea & Febiger, 1980
11. Frankel VH, Burstein AH: *Orthopaedic Biomechanics*—the Application of Engineering to the Musculoskeletal System. Philadelphia, PA, Lea & Febiger,1970
12. Smith, L.K., Weiss, E.L. & Lehmkuhl, L.D. (1996). *Brunnstrom's clinical kinesiology* (5th ed.). Philadelphia: F.A. Davis.

BIOMECHANICS OF UPPER LIMB

SHOULDER COMPLEX

The shoulder complex is composed of:

1. Glenohumeral (GH) Joint.
2. Sternoclavicular (SC) Joint.
3. Acromioclavicular (AC) Joint.
4. Scapulothoracic (ST) Joint.

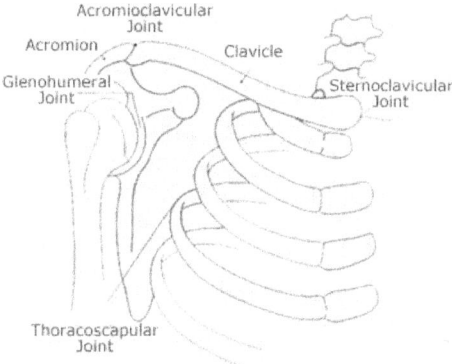

Glenohumeral Joint:

Articulation between head of the humerus and glenoid cavity of the scapula.

Synovial, ball and socket joint.

Capsules surrounds the joint and is attached medially to the margin of the glenoid cavity outside the labrum; laterally it is attached to the anatomic neck of the humerus.

Ligaments:

- Coracohumeral ligament:
    - ✓ Limits external rotation.
    - ✓ Anterior band elongates with and limits GH Extension
    - ✓ Posterior band elongates with and limits GH Flexion
- Glenohumeral ligament:
    - Once the glenohumeral joint is externally rotated, this ligament elongates with and limits abduction.

Synovial Membrane lines the capsule and is attached to the margins of the cartilage covering the articular surfaces.

Nerve Supply: Axillary and Suprascapular nerves.

Bursae:

Several bursae are associated with the shoulder complex, all contribute to function, the most important are the subacromial and subdeltoid bursae.

These bursae separate the supraspinatus tendon and the head of the humerus from the acromion, coracoid process, coracoacromial ligament, and deltoid muscle. The bursae may be separate but are commonly continuous with each other. The subacromial bursa permits smooth gliding between the humerus and supraspinatus tendon and its surrounding structures.

Glenohumeral Motions:

The GH joint is usually described as having 3° of freedom:

Movement	Location	Magnitude
Flexion	Saggital Plane Coronal Axis	$0°-120°$
Extension	Saggital Plane Coronal Axis	$0°-50°$
Abduction	Coronal Plane Saggital Axis	$0°-90°$
Adduction	Coronal Plane Saggital Axis	$90°-0°$
Internal Rotation	Transverse Plane Vertical Axis	$0°-70°$
External Rotation	Transverse Plane Vertical Axis	$0°-90°$

Arthrokinematics of the glenohumeral joint during glenohumeral abduction:

- Convex humeral head rolls upward and glides downward on scapula's concave glenoid fossa.
- Humerus' greater tubercle will impinge on the coracoacromial ligament or the acromion process unless the humerus externally rotates.
- Forces that guide the arthrokinematics:
    1. glenohumeral ligament
    2. **rotator cuff muscles**

Close-packed positions of the GH joint:

1. Horizontal Abduction and External Rrotation
2. Flexion and Internal Rotation

Scapulohumeral Rhythm:

The combination of concomitant Gleno Humeral and ScapuloThoracic motion is most commonly referred to as scapulohumeral rhythm. The complete range of shoulder flexion and abduction is 180° out of which 120 ° of movement occurs at GH joint and 60° of movement occurs at ST joint. Thus, overall ratio is 2° of GH motion to1 ° of ST motion. Later modified by Mc Millan (1966) to Scapulohumeroclavicular rhythm as clavicle participates along with the scapula and humerus. However, the appropriate terminology to describe the movement of the whole complex would be **"Scapulohumeroclaviculothoracic rhythm"**. In total 180 of elevation contribution of GH joint is 120 while the rest 60 through outward rotation of the scapula i.e, ratio 2:1. For every 15 of arm abduction, 10 take place at GHJoint while rest 5 by rotation of scapula upon thorax. Out of 60 of scapular rotation, 30 due to elevation of clavicle at SC Joint and remaining 30 at AC Joint.

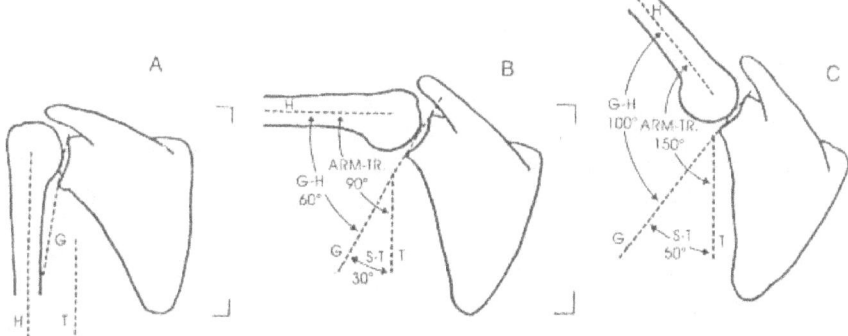

Scapulohumeral rhythm serves at least two purposes.

1. It preserves the length-tension relationships of the glenohumeral muscles; the muscles do not shorten as much as they would without the scapula's upward rotation, and so can sustain their force production through a larger portion of the range of motion.
2. It prevents impingement between the humerus and the acromion. Because of the difference in size between the glenoid fossa and the humeral head, subacromial impingement can occur unless relative movement between the humerus and scapula is limited. Simultaneous movement of the humerus and scapula during shoulder elevation limits relative (arthrokinematic) movement between the two bones.

Muscles of the shoulder girdle

(Classified into three groups according to location of attachments)

I. FROM AXIAL SKELETON TO SHOULDER GIRDLE (SCAPULA AND CLAVICLE)
   - Serratus anterior
   - Upper trapezius
   - Middle trapezius
   - Lower trapezius
   - Rhomboideus major and minor
   - Pectoralis minor

- Levator Scapulae

II. FROM SCAPULA AND CLAVICLE TO HUMERUS
- Deltoid
- "Rotator cuff"
  - supraspinatus
  - infraspinatus
  - teres minor
  - subscapularis
- Teres major
- Coracobrachialis
- Biceps brachii (long head)
- Triceps brachii (long head)

III. FROM AXIAL SKELETON TO HUMERUS
- Pectoralis major
- Latissimus dorsi

SHOULDER STABILITY

The shoulder is stabilised by both **static** and **dynamic** stabilisers, which work in synchrony to maintain shoulder stability.

STATIC STABILISERS
A) Vacuum Effect There are three mechanisms providing the vacuum effect. These are:
1. **Intracapsular pressure** - This is normally a negative pressure within the shoulder joint. Perforation of the joint breaks that pressure thus leading to slight excess in mobility of the joint. A slightly negative intra-articular pressure exists in a normal shoulder aids in centring the humeral head.
2. **Suction effect** - The glenoid labrum acts on the humeral head like a plunger.
3. **Adhesion cohesion** - when two wet surfaces, such as the humeral head and glenoid, come into contact with each other this creates an adhesion-cohesion bond, which provides stability to the glenohumeral articulation.

B) Glenoid : The upward tilt of glenoid fossa produce partial bony block against humeral inferior translation

The glenoid is normally retroverted 7 degrees to the scapula, but the scapula is anteverted 30 degrees to the coronal plane of the body, thus preventing **posterior instability**. .

C) Glenoid Labrum

The glenoid labrum is approximately 9mm thick, thus serves to deepen the glenoid socket. It conforms perfectly to the curvature of the humeral head and increases glenoid depth by 50%.).

D) Capsule

The glenohumeral joint capsule is thickened to form specific glenohumeral ligaments, the most significant of these is the **inferior** glenohumeral**ligament**. This forms a band anteriorly and posteriorly, the anterior band being the thicker of the two. These bands provide stability in internal and external rotation, with the anterior band tightening in external rotation and abduction, whilst the posterior tightens in internal rotation. Together they form a hammock inferiorly resisting inferior translation.

DYNAMIC STABILISERS
A) Proprioception

It has been shown that the glenohumeral joint capsule has numerous mechanoreceptors particularly within the anterior and inferior capsule (Jerosch 1997 and Gohlke 1998). In abduction and external rotation these mechanoreceptors are most likely activated as the humeral head comes into contact with the capsule sending a signal to the stabilising muscles of the shoulder providing containment and stability of the humeral head.

B) Muscles

The muscles of the shoulder are divided into the scapular muscles which transfer energy generated from the trunk and lower limbs into the arm and the rotator cuff muscles which are the fine tuning muscles maintaining the centre of rotation of the humeral head.

The rotator cuff muscles provide significant stability to the shoulder joint, almost hugging the joint to the glenoid.

The subscapularis muscle provides anterior stability when the arm is in neutral but less so as the arm comes into abduction (Turkel et al. 1984).

The infraspinatus and Teres minor act together to reduce the strain on the antero-inferior glenohumeral ligament in abduction and external rotation. They are therefore known as the "hamstrings" of the glenohumeral joint (Cain et al. 1987). The scapular muscles provide a stable base for shoulder movement. The key force couples in scapular mobility and stability are the lower trapezius and serratus anterior muscles, but the upper trapezius levator scapulae, rhomboids and pectoralis minor also provide stability and mobility. Repetitive or chronic scapular protraction may result in excessive strain, and ultimately, insufficiency in the anterior band of the IGHL (Weiser et al. 1999).

Gleno-humeral Force Couple:

- Supraspinatus fixes head of humerus to glenoid.
- Humeral head is maintained and stabilized in glenoid cavity by the downward pull of short rotators ie.,Infraspinatus,Subscapularis and teres minor.
- Head of humerus pulled into abduction by strong action of deltoid.

Scapulo-Humeral Force:

Acts as main force behind 60 degrees of outward rotation of scapula.

- Upper Trapezius acting on acromion rotates scapula outwards.
- Lower trapezius pull lower scapular spine carries outward rotation of scapula.
- Serratus anterior provide strongest force outward rotation of scapula.

Scapulothoracic (ST) joint

Articulation of the scapula with the thorax.

It is **not a true anatomic** joint.

Scapulothoracic Position:

Posterior thorax approximately 2 inches from the midline, between the second through seventh ribs.

30° to 40° forward of the frontal plane, tipped anteriorly approximately 10° to 20° from vertical.

Scapulothoracic Motions:

*Elevation / Depression.

* Protraction / Retraction (Abduction / Adduction).

*Upward Rotation / Downward Rotation (Medial Rotation / Lateral Rotation).

Elevation and **depression** - Scapula moves upward (cephalic) or downward (caudally) **Protraction** and **retraction** - scapula away from or toward the vertebral column.

Upward and **downward** rotations - movement of the inferior angle away from the vertebral column (upward rotation) or movement of the inferior angle toward the vertebral column (downward rotation).

Sternoclavicular Joint:

Articulation between the sternal end of the clavicle, manubrium sterni, and the first costal cartilage.

Synovial double – plane joint.

Capsule surrounds the joint and is attached to the margins of the articular surfaces.

Articular Disc: Flat fibrocartilaginous disc lies within the joint and divides the joint's interior into two compartments.

Ligaments:

1) Sternoclavicular (SC) Ligaments.

2) Costoclavicular Ligament

3) Interclavicular Ligament.

The anterior & posterior SC ligaments reinforce the capsule.

SC ligaments check anterior and posterior move head of the clavicle.

Costoclavicular ligament checks elevation of the clavicle.

Interclavicular ligament is present between the two clavicles and it check excessive depression or downward glide of the clavicle.

Synovial membrane lines the capsule and is attached to the margins of the cartilage covering the articular surfaces.

Nerve Supply: Supraclavicular nerve & nerve to subclavius.

Sternoclavicular Motions:

- Elevation 45^0 / Depression 15^0.
- Protraction 15^0 / Retraction 15^0.
- Anterior Rotation / Posterior Rotation 30^0 to 55^0.

Acromioclavicular Joint:

Articulation between the acromion of the scapula and the lateral end of the clavicle. It is Synovial plane joint.

Its **capsule** surrounds the joint and is attached to the margins of the articular surfaces.

A wedge-shaped fibrocartilaginous disc projects into the joint cavity from above.

Ligaments:

1) Acromioclavicular Ligaments.

2) Coracoclavicular Ligaments.

Superior and inferior acromioclavicular ligaments reinforce the joint capsule.

Coracoclavicular ligament is divided into a lateral portion, the trapezoid ligament, and a medial portion, the conoid ligament.

Both portions of the coracoclavicular ligament prevent upward rotation of the scapula at the AC joint.

Synovial membrane lines the capsule and is attached to the margins of the cartilage covering the articular surfaces.

Nerve Supply: Suprascapular Nerve.

Acromioclavicular Motions:

Medial Rotation / Lateral Rotation.

Anterior Tipping / Posterior Tipping.

Medial and lateral rotation of the scapula occurs around a vertical axis through the AC joint. Medial and lateral rotation brings the glenoid fossa medially (or anteriorly) and laterally (or posteriorly), respectively.

These motions must occur to maintain the contact of the scapula with the horizontal curvature of the thorax as the scapula slides around the thorax in protraction and retraction.

Coracoacromial Arch:

The coracoacromial (or suprahumeral) arch is formed by the coracoid process, the acromion, and the coracoacromial ligament.

The coracoacromial arch protects the structures beneath it from direct trauma from above which may occur through simple daily tasks as carrying a heavy bag slung over the shoulder. It also prevents the head of the humerus from dislocating superiorly. When the suprahumeral space is narrowed, the impingement of the supraspinatus tendon and subacromial bursa increases.

Refrences:

1. Nigg, B.M. and Herzog, W. (eds) (1999) *Biomechanics of the Musculoskeletal System*, Chichester: Wiley.
2. Frankel VH, Nordin M (eds): *Basic Biomechanics of the Skeletal System*. Philadelphia, PA, Lea & Febiger, 1980
3. P. Levangie, C. Norkin, 2000, *Joint Structure and Function: A Comprehensive Analysis*, F.A. Davis Company.
4. Knudson, D.V. and Morrison, C.S. (2002) *Qualitative Analysis of Human Movement*, 2nd edn, Champaign, IL: Human Kinetics.
5. Bartlett, R.M., Stockill, N.P., Elliott, B.C. and Burnett A.F. (1996) 'The biomechanics of fast bowling in men's cricket: a review', *Journal of Sports Science*, 14: 403–24.
6. Dave Thompson(2001) Retrieved from http://moon.ouhsc.edu/dthompso/namics/lecsked.htm
7. Robert A. Donatelli 2008, *Physical Therapy of the Shoulder*, Elsevier, Churchill Livingstone

ELBOW COMPLEX

Artculation between the trochlea and capitulum of the humerus and the trochlear notch of the ulna and the head of the radius. Synovial hinge joint.

Capsule: Anteriorly it is attached above to the humerus along the upper margins of the coronoid and radial fossae and to the front of the medial and lateral epicondyles and below to the margin of the coracoid process of the ulna and to the annular ligament, which surrounds the head of the radius.

Posteriorly it is attached above to the margins of the olecranon fossa of the humerus and below to the upper margin and sides of the olecranon process of the ulna and to the annular ligament.

Ligaments:

The two main ligaments associated with the elbow joints are the medial (ulnar) and lateral (radial) collateral ligaments.

The medial (ulnar) collateral ligament (MCL) is consists anterior band, posterior band, transverse band.

The lateral (radial) collateral ligament (LCL) is provide protection against varus stress in some positions of the elbow.

Synovial membrane lines the capsule and covers fatty pads in the floors of the coronoid, radial, and olecranon fossae; it is continuous below with the synovial membrane of the proximal radioulnar joint.

Nerve Supply: Branches from the median, ulnar, musculocutaneous, and radial nerves.

Axis of Motion: The axis for flexion and extension is relatively fixed and passes through the center of the trochlea and capitulum bisecting the longitudinal axis of the shaft of the humerus.

Carrying Angle:

When the upper extremity is in the anatomic position, the long axis of the humerus, and the long axis of the forearm form an acute angle medially when they meet at the elbow. The angulation is due to the configuration of the articulating surfaces and results in a normal valgus angulation of the forearm in relation to the humerus. This angle is called the **carrying angle** and is slightly greater in women than men.

The average angle in men is about 5°, whereas in women it is about 10° to 15°.

An increase in the carrying angle is considered to be abnormal, especially if it occurs unilaterally. When the angle is increased beyond the average, it is called **cubitus valgus**.

Range of Motion:

Flexion / Extension $0^0 - 146^0$

Superior Radioulnar Joints:

Articulation between the circumference of the head of the radius and the annular ligament and the radial notch on the ulna. It is Synovial pivot joint.

Capsule encloses the joint and is continuous with that of the elbow joint.

Ligaments: Three ligaments associated with the proximal radioulnar joint are the annular and quadrate ligaments and the oblique cord. The annular ligament is a strong band that encircles the radial head.

The quadrate ligament limits the spin of the radial head in supination and pronation.

Synovial membrane is continuous above with that of the elbow joint. Below it is attached to the inferior margin of the articular surface of the radius and the lower margin of the radial notch of the ulna.

Nerve Supply: Branches of the median, ulnar, musculocutaneous, and radial nerves.

Inferior Radioulnar Joint:

Articulation: Between the rounded head of the ulna and the ulnar notch on the radius.

Synovial pivot joint.

Capsule encloses the joint but is deficient superiorly.

Articular Disc:

This is triangular and composed of fibrocartilage. It is attached by its apex to the lateral side of the base of the styloid process of the ulna and by its base to the lower border of the ulnar notch of the radius. It shuts off the distal radioulnar joint from the wrist and strongly unites the radius to the ulna.

Ligaments:

The dorsal and palmar radioulnar ligaments, as well as the interosseous membrane, which stabilizes both proximal and distal joints, reinforce the distal radioulnar joint. The interosseous membrane is described simply as a broad collaginous sheet that runs between the radius and ulna. The fibres of the central band run distally and medially from the radius to the ulna.

Maximum strain in the fibres of the central band occurs when the forearm is in a neutral position (midway between supination & pronation).

The interosseous membrane provides stability for both the superior and inferior radioulnar joints.

When under tension, the membrane not only binds the joints together, but also provides for the transmission of forces from the hand and distal end of the radius to the ulna.

Synovial membrane lines the capsule passing from the edge of one articular surface to that of the other.

Nerve Supply: Anterior interosseous nerve and posterior interosseous nerve.

Axis of Motion: The axis of motion for pronation and supination is a longitudinal axis extending from the centre of the radial head to the centre of the ulnar head.

Range of Motion:

A total ROM of 150° has been ascribed to the radioulnar joints.

The range of motion of pronation and supination is assessed with the elbow in 90° of flexion. This position stabilizes the humerus so that radioulnar joint rotation may be distinguished from rotation that is occurring at the shoulder joint.

Arthrokinematics

Elbow and radio-ulnar arthrokinematics

Applying the rules of concavity and convexity to the humero-ulnar joint:

- In an Open Chain, concave ulnar surface rolls and glides in same direction on convex humeral surface.
- In a Closed Chain, the convex humeral surface rolls and glides in opposite directions on the concave ulnar surface.

During open chain elbow extension: ulna rolls and glides posteriorly on humerus while

- radius moves distally
- ulna and radius spread apart
- ulna and radius pronate with respect to each other.

Open chain elbow flexion: ulna rolls and glides anteriorly on humerus while

- radius moves proximally
- ulna and radius move closer together
- ulna and radius supinate with respect to each other.

Refrences:
1. Nigg, B.M. and Herzog, W. (eds) (1999) *Biomechanics of the Musculoskeletal System*, Chichester: Wiley.
2. Frankel VH, Nordin M (eds): Basic *Biomechanics of the Skeletal System*. Philadelphia, PA, Lea & Febiger, 1980
3. P. Levangie, C. Norkin, 2000, *Joint Structure and Function: A Comprehensive Analysis*, F.A. Davis Company.
4. Dave Thompson(2001) Retrieved from http://moon.ouhsc.edu/dthompso/namics/lecsked.htm
5. Knudson, D.V. and Morrison, C.S. (2002) *Qualitative Analysis of Human Movement*, 2nd edn, Champaign, IL: Human Kinetics.

WRIST COMPLEX

The wrist (carpus) consists of two compound joints: the radiocarpal and the midcarpal joints, referred to collectively as the wrist complex.

Axis and motions

Joint	Axis	Motion	Close-packed position
Wrist radio-carpal mid-carpal	Lateral	Flexion / Extension	Extension
	A-P	Ulnar and Radial deviation	

Normal ranges are 78° to 85° of flexion, 60° to 85° of extension, 15° to 21° of radial deviation, and 38° to 45° of ulnar deviation.

Radiocarpal Joint:

The radiocarpal joint is formed by the radius and radioulnar disc (triangularfibrocartilage complex [TFCC]) proximally and by scaphoid, lunate, and triquetrum distally.

The scaphoid, lunate, and triquetrum, pisiform compose the proximal carpal row. The pisiform functions entirely as a sesamoid bone, presumably to increase the moment arm (MA) of the flexor carpi ulnaris that attaches to it.

Midcarpal Joint:

The midcarpal joint is the articulation between the scaphoid, lunate, and triquetrum proximally and the distal carpal row composed of the trapezium, trapezoid, capitate, and hamate.

Together the bones of the distal carpal row contribute 2° of freedom to the wrist complex, with varying amounts of radial/ulnar deviation and flexion/extension credited to the joint..

The functional union of the distal carpals with each other and with their contiguous metacarpals not only serves the wrist complex, but also are the foundation for the transverse and longitudinal arches of the hand.

Ligaments of the Wrist Complex:

Extrinsic ligaments are those that connect the carpals to the radius or ulnar proximally or to the metacarpals distally.

Intrinsic ligaments are those that interconnect the carpals themselves and are also known as intercarpal or interosseous ligaments ..

Volar Carpal Ligaments:

The composite ligament known as the volar radiocarpal ligament has been described most commonly as having three distinct bands:

Radioscaphoid

Radiotriquetral

Radiocapitate

There are two intrinsic ligaments in the wrist complex, which are as follows:
- ✓ Scapholunate interosseous ligament
- ✓ Lunotriquetral interosseous ligament

Wrist arthrokinematics : In open chain movement, the convex surfaces of the scaphoid and lunate move on the concave surfaces of the radius and ulna.

- ➢ During flexion:
    - o scaphoid/lunate roll anteriorly (toward palm) and glide posteriorly (toward dorsum)
- ➢ During extension:

    scaphoid/lunate roll posteriorly(toward dorsum) and glide anteriorly (toward palm).
- ➢ During ulnar deviation:
    - o scaphoid/lunate roll toward ulna and glide toward radius.
- ➢ During radial deviation:
    - o scaphoid/lunate roll toward radius and glide toward ulna.

Muscles of the Wrist Complex:

Volar Wrist Musculature:

Six muscles have tendons crossing the volar aspect of the wrist and,therefore, are capable of creating a wrist flexion movement. These are as follows:

Palmaris Longus (PL)

Flexor Carpi Radialis (FCR)

Flexor Carpi Ulnaris (FCU)

Flexor Digitorum Superficialis (FDS)

Flexor Digitorum Profundus (FDP)

Flexor Pollicis Longus (FPL)

Dorsal Wrist Musculature:
- ✓ Extensor Carpi Radialis Longus (ECRL)
- ✓ Extensor Carpi Radialis Brevis (ECRB)
- ✓ Extensor Carpi Ulnaris (ECU)
- ✓ Extensor Digitorum Communis (EDC)
- ✓ Extensor Indicis Proprius (EIP)

- ✓ Extensor Digiti Minimi (EDM)
- ✓ Extensor Pollicis Longus (EPL)
- ✓ Extensor Pollicis Brevis (EPB)
- ✓ Abductor Pollicis Longus (APL)

Wrist Joint Pathology:

The flexed distal carpals glide dorsally on the lunate and triquetrum, accentuating the extension of the lunate and triquetrum. This zigzag pattern of the three segments (the scaphoid, the lunate and triquetrum, and the distal carpal row) is known as **dorsal intercalated segmental instability (DISI)**.

With sufficient ligamentous laxity, the capitate may sublux dorsally off the extended lunate and migrate into the gap between the flexed scaphoid and extended lunate. This deformity is called **scapholunate-advanced collapse (SLAC)**.

When the lunate is no longer linked with the triquetrum, the lunate and scaphoid together fall into flexion, and the triquetrum and distal carpal row extend. This ulnar perilunate instability is known as **volar intercalated segmental instability (VISI)**.

Three arches balance stability and mobility in the hand.
The proximal transverse arch is rigid, but the other two arches are flexible

1. PROXIMAL TRANSVERSE ARCH
2. DISTAL TRANSVERSE ARCH
3. LONGITUDINAL ARCH

The arches provide a balance between stability and mobility for grasping.

Joints of the hand

JOINT	STRUCTURE	AXIS	MOTION	CLOSE-PACKED POSITION
Metacarpo-phalangeal (MP)	Biaxial (condylar)	Lateral A-P	Flexion/Extension Abduction/Adduction	First: extension 2nd-5th: Flexion
Proximal Interphalangeal (PIP)	Uniaxial	Lateral	Flexion/Fxtension	Extension
Distal Interphalangeal (DIP)	uniaxial	lateral	flexion/extension	extension

- Metacarpophalangeal (MP)
    - condyloid, biaxial joints
    - joint's palmar aspect is palpable at level of distal palmar crease
    - proximal joint surface is convex and distal surface is concave

- roll and glide occur in same direction
  - anterior with flexion
  - posterior with extension.
- large metacarpal joint surface
- a fibrocartilaginous volar plate is lined with hyaline cartilage so that it augments or enlarges the proximal phalanx' relatively small articular surface.
- superficial to volar plate is the transverse metacarpal ligament
- joint capsule supported by two collateral ligaments
- close-packed position:
  - MP joints of digits 2 through 5: close-packed in flexion; we cannot abduct or adduct these joints when they are flexed.
  - MP joint of thumb: close-packed in extension
- Interphalangeal (IP)
  - uniaxial hinge joints
  - supported by two collateral ligaments, and by smaller versions of a volar plate.
  - Like MP joint, proximal joint surface is convex and distal surface is concave
    roll and glide occur in same direction
    - anterior with flexion
    - posterior with extension
  - close-packed in extension

EXTENSOR MECHANISM

The extensor mechanism is an elaboration of the extensor digitorum comunis (EDC) tendon on the dorsum of each phalanx. The extensor indicis (EI) and the extensor digiti minimi (EDM) insert into the extensor mechanisms of the second and fifth digits, respectively.

Several tendinous structures comprise the extensor mechanism:

EXTENSOR MECHANISM

1. EXTENSOR DIGITORUM TENDON
2. CENTRAL TENDON
3. LATERAL BANDS
4. HOOD REGION

1. The *EDC tendon* attaches by a tendinous slip to the proximal phalanx, through which it extends the MP joint.
2. The *central tendon* (or "slip") proceeds dorsally to attach to base of middle phalanx, where tension can extend the PIP joint.

3. the *lateral bands* proceed on either side of

4. the *extensor hood* surrounds the MP joint

dorsal midline and rejoin before attaching to the distal phalanx. Tension in the lateral bands extends the DIP joint. laterally, medially, and dorsally, and receives tendinous fibers from the lumbricales and interossei.

5. Fibers of the *oblique retinacular ligament* (ORL) attach at the sides of the proximal phalanx and digital tendon sheaths, and proceed to distal portion of lateral bands. Thus, the ORL's line of application is volar to the PIP joint's lateral axis and dorsal to the DIP joint's lateral axis.

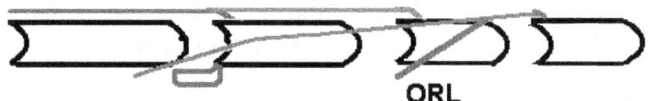

OBLIQUE RETINACULAR LIGAMENT (ORL)

PIP extension (produced by other tissues in the extensor mechanism) elongates the ORL, creating passive tension that extends the DIP. The DIP extension helps open the hand.

DIP flexion (produced by the FDP) elongates the ORL, creating passive tension that flexes the PIP. The PIP flexion assists in finger closure.

Prehension: Activities of hand involve grasping.

Power Grip (full hand prehension)-Cylindrical grip (holding glass), Spherical grip (holding cricket ball), Hook Grip(holding suitcase, bucket),Lateral Grip (holding a cigarette)

Precision Grip (finger-thumb prehension)-Pad-to-Pad prehension,Tip-to-Tip prehension,Pad-to-Side prehension

Wrist Functional Position: Extn.20^0,Ulnar deviation 10^0,Flexed at MP Joint 45^0,PIP 30^0 slightly fled at DIP joints.

Refrences:

1. Nigg, B.M. and Herzog, W. (eds) (1999) *Biomechanics of the Musculoskeletal System*, Chichester: Wiley.
2. Frankel VH, Nordin M (eds): *Basic Biomechanics of the Skeletal System.*Philadelphia, PA, Lea & Febiger, 1980
3. P. Levangie , C. Norkin,2000, *Joint Structure and Function: A Comprehensive Analysis*, F.A. Davis Company.
4. Knudson, D.V. and Morrison, C.S. (2002) *Qualitative Analysis of Human Movement*, 2nd edn, Champaign, IL: Human Kinetics
5. Dave Thompson(2001) Retrieved from http://moon.ouhsc.edu/dthompso/namics/lecsked.htm
6. Hertling, D., & Kessler, R. M. (1996). *Management of common musculoskeletal disorders: Physical therapy principles and methods*. (3rd ed.).Philadelphia: J.B. Lippincott.
7. Smith, L.K., Weiss, E.L. & Lehmkuhl, L.D.(1996). *Brunnstrom's clinical kinesiology*. (5th ed.). Philadelphia: F.A. Davis.

BIOMECHANICS OF LOWER LIMB
HIP COMPLEX

The hip joint is formed by the articulation of the head of the femur into the acetabulum of the pelvis.

Ball-and-socket joint. Synovial joint

The acetabulum is formed by the pubis, ischium and ilium bones.

Angle of Acetabulam
- ✓ Acetabulam is oriented at the lateral side of each pelvic bone.
- ✓ It is also directed somewhat inferiorly and anteriorly.
- ✓ The magnitude of inferior orientation can be assesed by using a line connecting the lateral rim of the acetabulam and the center of the femoral head this line forms an angle with the verticle known as the **Center Edge Angle**.
- ✓ The magnitude of the anterior orientation of the acetabulam may be referred to as the angle of acetabular anteversion.

Joint Capsule
- ✓ Strong and dense.
- ✓ It covers the femoral head and neck and attaches to the base of the neck.
- ✓ It has a two sets of fibers.
- ✓ Circular fibers form a collar around a femoral neck called the zona orbicularis.
- ✓ The longitudinal fiber are retinacular fibers deep in the capsule that travel along the neck toward the femoral head.
- ✓ Retinacular fibers carry blood vessels arise from the vascular ring located at the base of neck and formed by the medial & lateral circumflex femoral arteries (branches of the deep femoral artery).

Angle of Inclination (Between the femoral neck and shaft)

The angle of inclination is measured in the frontal plane and typically ranges from 115^0 to 140^0 degrees.

Coxa Vara:

An angle between femoral neck and shaft less than $115°$; increases stress on femoral neck. This:

1. Shortens the limb;

2. Decreases the effectiveness of the abductors;
3. Increases the load on the femoral neck;
4. Reduces the load on the femoral head.

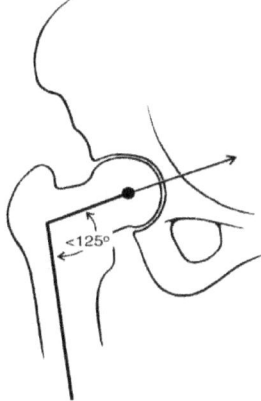

Fig. coxa vara

Coxa Valga:

- ✓ An angle between femoral neck and shaft greater than 140°; increases pressure into the joint
- ✓ This:
  1. Lengthens the limb;
  2. Mimics contracture of the hip abductors;
  3. Reduces the load on the femoral neck;

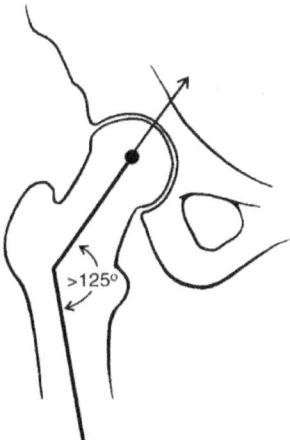

fig. Coxa valga

Angle of Torsion:

The angle between the axis of the neck and the transverse axis that passes through the femoral condyles.

a) Normal 12°-14°
b) Anteversion >15°
c) Retroversion <12°

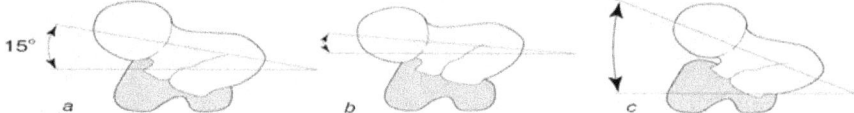

Excessive Anteversion :

- An increase in the angle of torsion (anteversion) influences the rotation of the limb and produces a **toe in gait (pigeon toes)**.

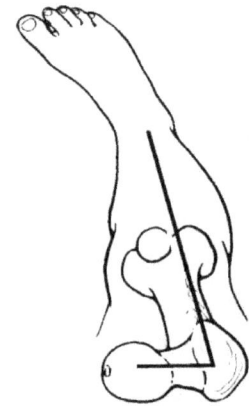

Fig. Excessive Anteversion

Retroversion:

- A decrease in the angle of torsion (retroversion) influences the rotation of the limb and produces a **toe out gait (duck feet)**.

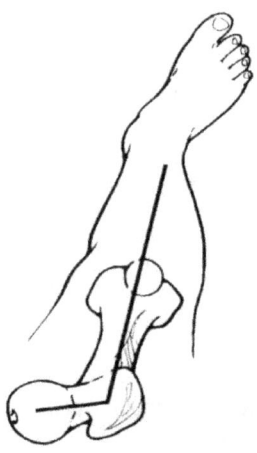

Fig. Retroversion

Ligaments of the Hip Joint

Ligament Name	Location	Function*
Iliofemoral "Y"	Ant. Surf. Capsule	Prevents hyperextension during standing
Pubofemoral	Ant. & Inf. Surf. Cap	Limits abduction and extension
Ischiofemoral	Posterior Surf. Capsule	Prevents hyperextension
Lig. of Head	Intracapsular - betw. fem. head and acetab. notch	Weak, contains artery, may limit adduction
Transverse Acetab.	Continuation of acetab. labrum over notch	Helps hold head in acetabular fossa

Hip Joint Innervation:

- ✓ Proprioception, Pain and Vasomotor fibers by nerves supplying prime movers of joint.
- ✓ Ant - Femoral n. and Obturator n.
- ✓ Post – Small branches from sacral plexus
    - o (N. to Quad. Femoris; Sup. Gluteal n.)

Hip Joint – Blood Supply

Med. & Lat. Fem. Circumflex a.; Acetabular artery. (30%)

Muscles:

- External rotators: piriformis, quadratus femoris, Obturator internus and externus, gemellus superior and inferior,
- Flexors: iliopsoas, rectus femoris
- Adductors: adductor magnus, adductor longus and brevis, pectineus, gracilis
- Internal rotators: gluteus medius, gluteus minimus, tensor fascia latae
- Extensors: semitendinosus and semimembranosus, biceps femoris, gluteus maximus
- Abductors: gluteus medius, gluteus minimus

Movements

- **Flexion**- iliopsoas muscle, sartorius, rectus femoris, pectineus
- **Extension**- guteus maximus, hamstrings
- **Adduction**- adductor longus, brevis, magnus, gracilis
- **Abduction**- gluteus medius and gluteus minimus
- **Lateral rotation**- gluteus maximus, quadratus femoris, piriformis, obturator internus and externus, gemelli

- **Medial rotation-** glueteus minimus and medius, tensor fasciae latae

R.O.M

- Varies with age, sex
- Flexion 120–135 degrees with knee flexed 90 degrees
- Extension 0–15 degrees
- Abduction 0–30 degrees
- Rotation generally 45 degrees in each direction (more LR with males, more MR with females)
- AXES OF MOTION

JOINT	AXIS	MOTION	CLOSE-PACKED POSITION
Hip	Lateral	Flex/Ext	combined Extension, Internal Rotation, and Abduction
	AP	Abd/Add	
	Longitudinal	ER/IR	

HIP ARTHROKINEMATICS

In an open chain, when the convex femoral head moves on a stationary acetabulum,

FLEXION	femoral head rolls anteriorly and glides posteriorly on acetabulum
EXTENSION	femoral head rolls posteriorly and glides anteriorly
ABDUCTION	femoral head rolls laterally and glides medially
ADDUCTION	femoral head rolls medially and glides laterally

Weight bearing structures of the hip joint

- The weight bearing lines of both the pelvis and the femur are evident by the arrangement of trabeculae. There are two major system-Medial trabeculae system and Lateral trabeculae system. The medial trabeculae system, conciding with cortical bone on the medial shaft of the femur, help in resist the compressive forces on the inside of the bending stresses of the shaft. The lateral trabeculae system, conciding with lateral cortical bone, help to resist the tensile forces on the outside of the bending stresses on the shaft. An area in the femoral neck where the trabeculae are relatively thin and do not cross each other, called as the **Zone of weakness**.

Lumbar pelvic motion:

- When the femur, pelvis, and spine move together in a coordinated manner to produce a larger ROM than might be available to one segment alone, the hip joint is participating in an open chain and the term lumbar –pelvic motion is used.

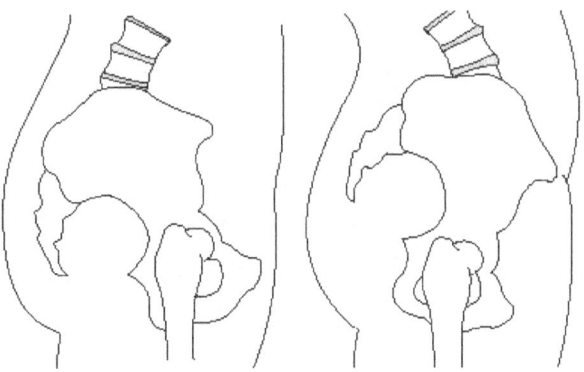

Fig. Posterior Pelvic & Anterior Pelvic Tilt

Posterior Pelvic Tilt: Symphysis pubis moves superiorly and lumbar spine flexes slightly, hip joint is extends.

Anterior Pelvic Tilt: Symphysis pubis moves inferiorly and lumbar spine extends, hip joint flexes.

Lateral Pelvic Tilt: Occur either as hip hiking or as pelvic drop (drop of opposite side of the pelvis).

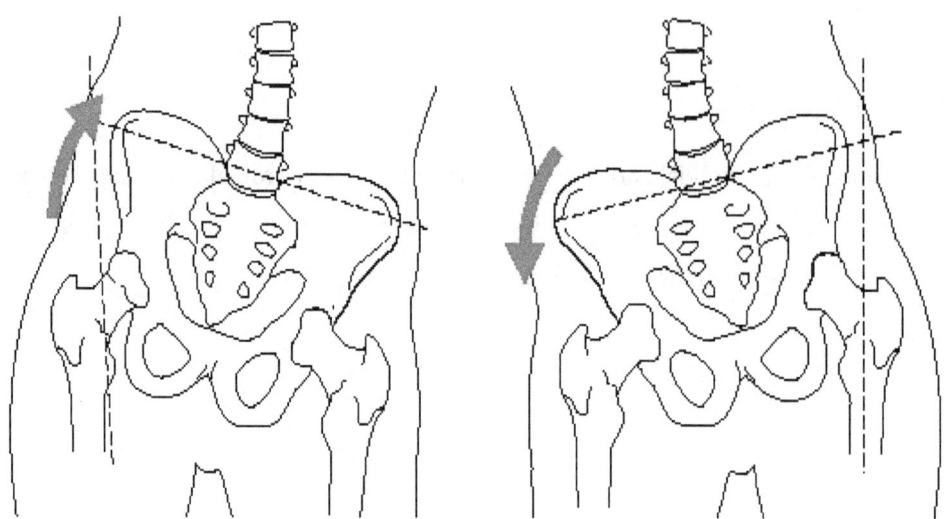

Fig. **Lateral Pelvic Tilt**

Forward Pelvic Rotation: Forward rotation of the pelvis occur when the side of the pelvis opposite to supporting hip joint moves anteriorly.

Backward Pelvic Rotation: Backward rotation of the pelvis occur when the side of the pelvis opposite to supporting hip joint moves posteriorly.

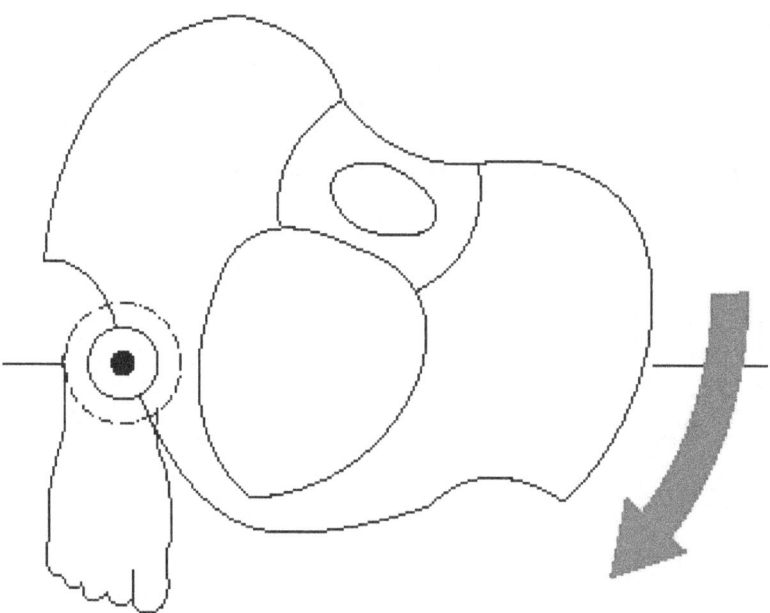

Fig. Rotation of Pelvis and Hip Transverse Plane

Muscle function in stance

Bilateral stance-

- Weight are evenly distributed.
- Both the hip are in slight hyperextension position.
- The LOG falls posteriorly to the hips.
- This LOG causes extension moment force on the hips & tends to tilt the pelvis posteriorly on the femoral heads.
- During bilateral stance phase the weight of the superimposed body is transmitted through the sacroiliac joints along the pelvic trabeculae system to the right and left femoral heads.
- It is typically presumed that the weight of superimposed body weight HAT is 2/3 of the body weight.
- So that each femoral head receive ½ of the total body weight.
  Weight of the body acting equally around the right hip tends to drop the pelvis down on the left, whereas the weight acting around the left hip tends to drop the pelvis down on the right.

Unilateral stance

- The superimposed body weight is being supported by a single limb.
- The supported leg carry full burden of the body weight, not the hanging one.
- So the previously assumed 2/3 of body weight is carried by the supported leg.
- Additionally the weight of the unsupported leg with weight of HAT.
- The nonsupported limb must account half of the 1/3 portion of the body weight or the 1/6 of the full body weight.
- The force of gravity acting on HAT in the non weight bearing lower limb (HATLL) will create an adduction torque around the supporting hip joint ; gravity will attempt to drop the pelvis around the right weight bearing hip joint axis.

COMPENSATORY LATERAL LEAN OF THE TRUNK

- If there is a need to reduce the torque of gravity in unilateral stance and if the body weight cannot be reduced, the MA of the gravitational force can be reduced by laterally leaning the trunk over the pelvis toward the painful or weakness side.

- The compensatory lateral lean of the trunk toward the painful stance limb will swing's the LOG closer to the hip joint, there by reducing the gravitational MA.

Gravity's effect on hip joint movement during standing

In normal standing posture, the center of gravity of the mass superincumbent to the hip joint is located so that its line of application passes posterior to the hip joint's lateral axis (Kendall, McCreary, & Provance, 1993).

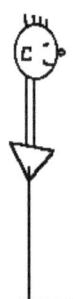

Gravity's force, acting at a distance from the axis of the hip joint, produces a posterior pelvic tilt. In a closed chain, with the femur relatively fixed, a posterior pelvic tilt produces hip extension. Hip flexor muscle activity controls gravity's hip extensor moment

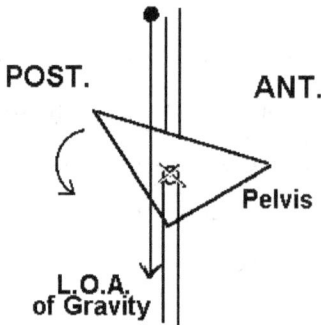

The idea that we activate muscles that oppose gravity's moment makes sense in terms of rotational equilibrium. But In this case, we need not use muscles to stabilize the hip joint during normal quiet standing, because an anterior ligament exists with the same line of application.

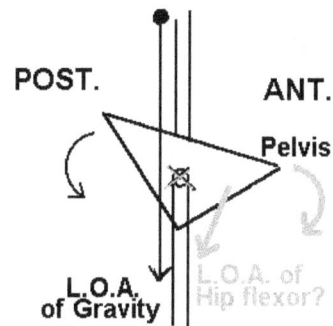

When the iliofemoral ligament elongates, like a very tight spring, it develops an elastic force. Although this force is passive, not active like a muscle's force, it is nevertheless directed at its points of attachment on the ilium and femur. The force prevents the attachments from being pulled further apart, that is, it prevents extension. A vector that represents this ligamentous force looks exactly like the one that depicts the force developed in a hip flexor muscle.

Assistive device helps people control the pelvis without developing large forces in the abductor muscles :

The secret in using an assistive device, like a cane, is to create an additional force that keeps the pelvis level in the face of gravity's tendency to adduct the hip during unilateral stance. The cane's force must substitute for the hip abductors.

A force that levels the pelvis efficiently, because its moment arm is relatively long, is directed upward from a point of application on the pelvis (vector C). The force originates on the side opposite the hip whose abductor muscles (vector M) are weak .

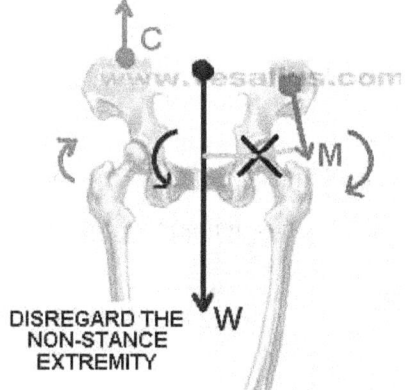
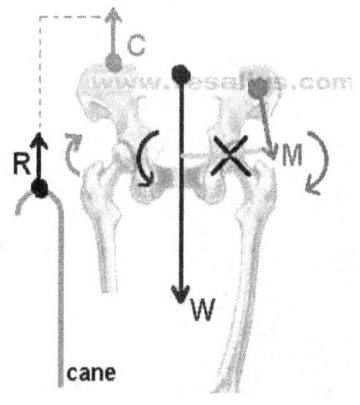

To produce a force like vector C with a cane, one must push the cane firmly into the ground in a vertical direction. Doing so generates an upward reaction force (vector R) whose magnitude equals the downward force one exerts on the cane.

Additionally, the person needs adequate strength in the muscles of the wrist, elbow, shoulder girdle, and trunk, whose effect is symbolized by the dashed line that connects vectors R and C. If not, he or she cannot efficiently transfer the cane's vertical reaction force (vector R) to the top of the pelvis (vector C) where it is needed.

Use of cane ipsilaterally

- Use of a cane on the side of pain or weakness would reduce the superimposed body weight by the amount of the downward thrust.
- The proportion of body weight that passes through the cane will not passes through the hip Suggests that it is realistic to accept that some one can push down on cane with approximately 15% of his body weight.
- It is not as effective in reducing hip joint compression.
- joint and will not create an adduction torque around the supporting hip joint.

Use of a cane contralaterally

- Use of cane in contralateral side opposite to side of pain ,or weak hip joint the reduction in HATLL is the same as it is when the cane is use in the same side as the painful hip joint.
- In addition to relieving some of the superimposed body weight ,the cane is in now position to assist the abductor muscles in providing a countertorque to the torque of gravity .

Compensation for muscle weakness

Because hip abductor activity is necessary to stabilize the hip in the frontal plane during unilateral stance, including the stance phase of walking, people with hip abductor weakness (note the relatively short vector M in the figure below) have a problem.

We might see the pelvis drop on the unsupported side if we ask a person to stand briefly on the limb whose hip abductors are weak. The, inability to maintain a level pelvis in unilateral stance is called a positive Trendelenburg sign.

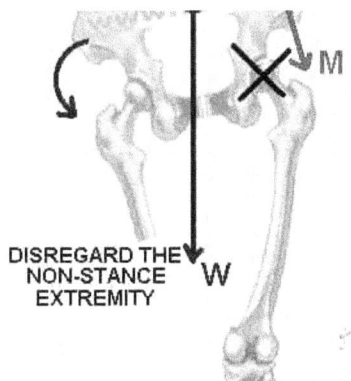

The most direct way to reorient the line of application of the gravity vector (note how vector W has shifted to the right), and so to shorten its moment arm with respect to the hip joint, is to lean the trunk toward the side of the hip whose abductor muscles are weak. This characteristic way of walking, in which the person leans laterally during stance, is sometimes called a Trendelenburg gait pattern or a gluteus medius limp.

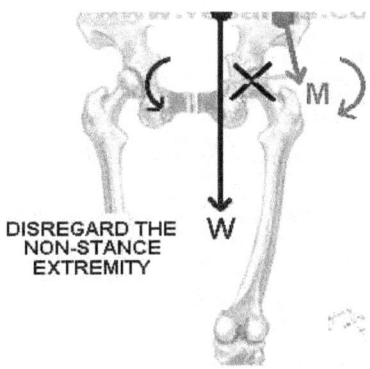

Refrences:

1. Adkins, S. B., Figler, R A. (2001). Hip pain in athletes. *American Family Physician*, 61:2109-2118.
2. Amendola, A., Wolcott, M. (2002). Bony injuries around the hip. *Sports Medicine and Arthroscopy Review*, 10:163-167.
3. Apkarian, J., et al. (1989). Three-dimensional kinematic and dynamic model of the lower limb. *Journal of Biomechanics*, 22:143-155
4. Blazevich, A. J. (2000). Optimizing hip musculature for greater sprint running speed. *NSCA Strength and Conditioning Journal,* 22:22-27.
5. Brown, L. P., Yavarsky, P. (1987). Locomotor biomechanics and pathomechanics: A review. *Journal of Orthopaedic and Sports Physical Therapy*, 9:3-10.
6. Knudson, D.V. and Morrison, C.S. (2002) *Qualitative Analysis of Human Movement*, 2nd edn, Champaign, IL: Human Kinetics.
7. Payton and R. Bartlett (eds) *Biomechanical Analysis of Movement in Sport and Exercise: The British Association of Sport and Exercise Sciences Guide*, Oxon: Routledge.
8. Nigg, B.M. and Herzog, W. (eds) (1999) *Biomechanics of the Musculoskeletal System*, Chichester: Wiley.
9. Frankel VH, Nordin M (eds*): Basic Biomechanics of the Skeletal System*.Philadelphia, PA, Lea & Febiger, 1980
10. P. Levangie , C. Norkin,2000, *Joint Structure and Function: A Comprehensive Analysis*, F.A. Davis Company.

KNEE JOINT

- 3 bones make up the knee joint Femur, Patella, Tibia
- Functionally = Modified hinge joint, Bi axial
- It is more complicated than a simple hinge joint due to some rotation that occurs to allow flexion and extension
- Fibula is non weightbearing / non articulating in the knee joint

The articulation between the femur and patella is a plane joint where the patella glides on the femur.

Femur: longest bone in body, distal end are medial and lateral condyles, the medial condyle is longer from front to back than the lateral condyle.

- This is what causes the rotation at the tibia in full extension.

Tibia: Tibial Tuberosity is where the patellar tendon attaches. Tibial Plateau is where the menisci are located.

- Patella: Largest sesamoid bone in the body
- Functions: Increase angle of pull of quads, Decrease friction between quad and condyles, acts as bony shield to protect condyles, Improves aesthetic appearance of knee.

Menisci (plural): Fibrocartilage disks that sit on tibial plateau.

- Medial is "C" shaped
- Lateral is "O" shaped
- Functions: Increases stability of the joint, cushions stresses.
- Blood supply to menisci: Inner 2/3 is avascular (no blood supply), Outer 1/3 does have blood supply.

Axis of motion

JOINT	AXIS	MOTION	CLOSE-PACKED POSITION
Tibio-Femoral Patello-Femoral	Lateral Longitudinal	Flexion/Extension Tibial Rotation	Extension

LIGAMENTS OF THE KNEE

1. medial collateral ligament (MCL)
2. lateral collateral ligament (LCL)
3. anterior cruciate ligament (ACL)

4. posterior cruciate ligament (PCL)

MCL	RESISTS VALGUS STRESS/FORCE
LCL	RESISTS VARUS STRESS/FORCE
MCL LCL PCL ACL	RESIST/LIMIT EXTENSION

TIBIO-FEMORAL ARTHROKINEMATICS

Viewed in the sagittal plane, the femur's articulating surface is convex while the tibia's in concave. We can predict arthrokinematics based on the rules of concavity and convexity:

DURING KNEE EXTENSION		DURING KNEE FLEXION	
OPEN CHAIN	CLOSED CHAIN	OPEN CHAIN	CLOSED CHAIN
TIBIA GLIDES ANTERIORLY ON FEMUR	FEMUR GLIDES POSTERIORLY ON TIBIA	TIBIA GLIDES POSTERIORLY ON FEMUR	FEMUR GLIDES ANTERIORLY ON TIBIA
from 20° knee flexion to full extension		from full knee extension to 20° flexion	
Tibia rotates externally	Femur rotates internally on stable tibia	Tibia rotates internally	Femur rotates externally on stable tibia

THE "SCREW-HOME" MECHANISM

Rotation between the tibia and femur occurs automatically between full extension (0°) and 20° of knee flexion. These figures illustrate *the top of the right tibial* plateau as we look down on it during knee motion.

DURING KNEE EXTENSION, the tibia glides anteriorly on the femur.	During the last 20 degrees of knee extension, anterior tibial glide persists on the tibia's medial condyle because its articular surface is longer in that dimension than the lateral condyle's.	Prolonged anterior glide on the medial side produces external tibial rotation, the "screw-home" mechanism.

THE SCREW-HOME MECHANISM REVERSES DURING KNEE FLEXION

When the knee begins to flex from a position of full extension, posterior tibial glide begins first on the longer medial condyle.	Between 0 deg. extension and 20 deg. of flexion, posterior glide on the medial side produces relative tibial internal rotation, a reversal of the screw-home mechanism.	

Muscles:

Quad muscles: Made up of 4 muscles: Vastus Medialis, Vastus intermedius, Vastus Lateralis, Rectus Femoris

- Vastus Medialis Oblique helps to keep the patella from subluxing laterally.
- Hamstrings: Made up of 3 muscles: Semitendinosus, Semimembranosus, Biceps femoris

Knee Joint Motion: Flexion: 130-140 degree, Extension 5-10 degrees

Patellofemoral Joint

- ✓ Articulation of the patella and femur
- ✓ Patella is a true sesamoid bone
- ✓ Posterior surface of the patella is covered with thick hyaline cartilage
- ✓ The patella slides within the trochlear groove

Q-angle:

The Q-angle is the angle formed by a line from the anterior superior spine of the ilium to the middle of the patella and a line from the middle of the patella to the tibial tuberosity.

Males typically have Q-angles between 10^0 to 14°, females between $15-17^o$.

Patella Alta: Patella shifts superiorly.

Patella Baja: Patella shifts inferiorly.

Crossed Eye Patella: Patella superior medial pole faces medially and inferior pole faces laterally.

Grass Hoppers Eye Patella: Patella faces upward and outward.

Refrences:

1. Nigg, B.M. and Herzog, W. (eds) (1999) *Biomechanics of the Musculoskeletal System*, Chichester: Wiley.
2. Frankel VH, Nordin M (eds): *Basic Biomechanics of the Skeletal System*.Philadelphia, PA, Lea & Febiger, 1980
3. P. Levangie, C. Norkin,2000, *Joint Structure and Function: A Comprehensive Analysis*, F.A. Davis Company.
4. Davies, G. J., et al. (1980). Knee examination. *Physical Therapy*, 60:1565-1574.
5. Knudson, D.V. and Morrison, C.S. (2002) *Qualitative Analysis of Human Movement*, 2nd edn, Champaign, IL: Human Kinetics.
6. Dave Thompson(2001) Retrieved from http://moon.ouhsc.edu/dthompso/namics/lecsked.htm
7. Blackburn, T A., Craig, E. (1980). Knee anatomy: A brief review. *Physical Therapy*, 60:1556-1560
8. Open versus closed chain kinetic exercises after anterior cruciate ligament reconstruction. A prospective randomized study. *The American Journal of Sports Medicine*, 23:401-406
9. Chesworth, B. M., et al. (1989). Validation of outcome measures in patients with patellofemoral syndrome. *Journal of Sports Physical Therapy*, 10(8):302-308
10. Hertling, D., & Kessler, R.M. (1996). *Management of common musculoskeletal disorders: Physical therapy principles and methods* (3rd ed.). Philadelphia: J.B.Lippincott.
11. Kendall, F.P., McCreary, E.K., & Provance, P.G. (1993). *Muscles: Testing and function* (4th ed.). Baltimore: Williams & Wilkins.

QUICK REVIEW OF BIOMECHANICS

FOOT & ANKLE:

STABILITY FUNCTIONS:
- ✓ Stable base of support for the body
- ✓ Rigid lever for effective push off during gait

MOBILTY DEMANDS:
- ✓ Dampening of rotations imposed by prox. joints
- ✓ Absorb shock
- ✓ Conform the foot to changing &varying terrain on which the foot is placed.

COMPONENTS:
- ▶ 28 BONES:

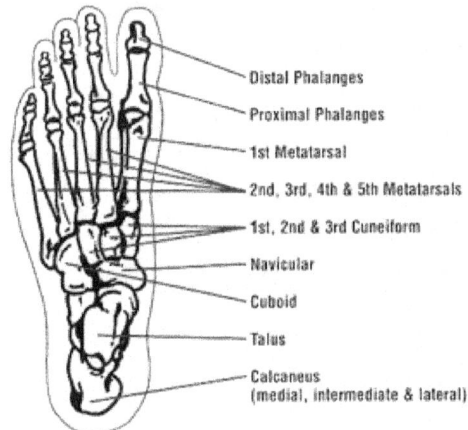

25 JOINTS
- ✓ Proximal & distal TF
- ✓ Ankle joints
- ✓ Subtalar joint
- ✓ Talonavicular & calcanecuboid joints
- ✓ 5 TMT joints
- ✓ 5 MTP joints
- ✓ 9 IP joints

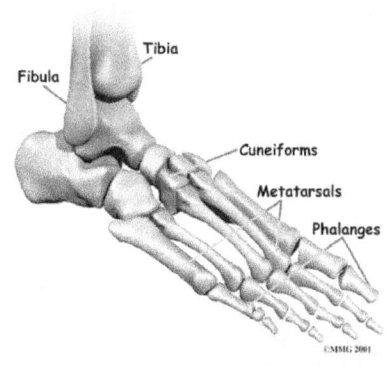

FUNCTIOAL SEGMENTS:

HIND FOOT = Talus, Calcaneum

MID FOOT = Navicular, Cuboid, 3 cuneiform

FOREFOOT = Metatarsal, Phalanges

ANKLE JOINT

ARTICULATION:
- ✓ Talocrural joint:
- ✓ Talus and distal tibia
- ✓ Talus and fibula

TYPE OF JOINT: synovial hinge joint

AXIS AND MOVEMENTS: single axis with 1^0 of freedom : dorsiflexion & plantarflexion

STRUCTURE OF THE ANKLE JOINT

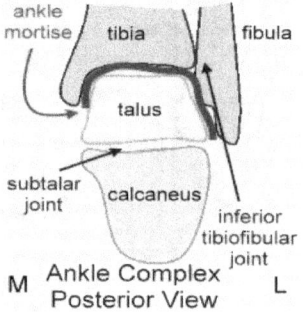

Proximal and distal TF joints
- ✓ Anatomically distinct from the ankle joint,
- ✓ Function exclusively to serve the ankle

STABILITY:
- ✓ Capsule: thin & weak ant. & post
- ✓ Ligaments:-
    1. Medial collateral ligament (deltoid ligament)
    2. Lateral collateral ligament

▶ Non weight bearing:

Pronation:
- ✓ DF of foot (saggital plane)

- ✓ Eversion (frontal plane)
- ✓ Abduction (transverse plane)

Supination:
- ✓ PF
- ✓ Inversion
- ✓ Adduction

ROM:

Weight bearing foot total range 40 degree (20 DF & 20 PF)

Non weight bearing range is 42 (23 and 23 respectively PF and DF)

SUBTALAR JOINT

- ✓ composite joint
- ✓ 3 separate plane articulation between talus sup.& calcaneus inf.
- ✓ triplanar movement around a single joint axis

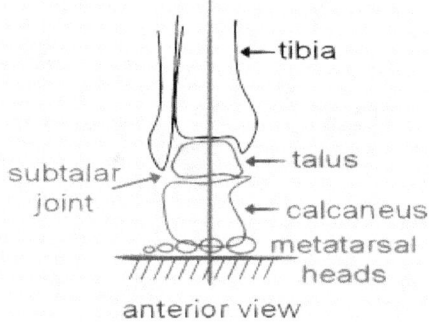

JOINT STRUCTURE

- ✓ Posterior talocalcaneal articulation
- ✓ Anterior and middle talocalcaneal articulation
- ▶ JOINT STABILITY:

Capsule:

Post. articulation : own capsule

Ant. & middle articulation: share capsule with TN joint

LIGAMENTS:

Ligamentous structure that support the ankle

- ✓ Calcaneofibular ligament
- ✓ Lateral talocalcaneal ligament
- ✓ Interosseus talocalcaneal ligament
- ✓ Cervical ligament
- ✓ Interosseus TCL

SUBTALAR JOINT FUNCTION

Arthrokinematics: Concave convex rule:

Post.articulation: Talus slides in the same direction

Ant. & middle articulation: Talar surface glides in the opp. Direction

Subtalar joint axis: inclined 42 degree upward & anteriorly from transverse plane (with a broad inter indiviudual range of 29-47) inclined medially 10 degree from saggital plane (with again head inter individual range of 8-24)

▶ Non weight bearing subtalar joint motion

Supination

Calcaneal motions of

1. adduction (vertical axis)
2. inversion (AP axis)
3. plantar flexion (coronal axis)

Pronation: vice versa

Weight bearing subtalar joint motion:

Supination:

- ✓ Calcaneus: inversion
- ✓ Talus: plantar flexion
- ✓ Tibia: medial rotation

Pronation: vice versa

TALOCALCANEONAVICULAR JOINT

Articulation of talus with navicular

TCN joint structure

Ties together Talonavicular & subtalar joints

Articulation: Proximally anterior portion of head of talus. Distally by concave posterior navicular.

Type of joint: ball and socket

Ligaments:

Spring ligament

Superomedial calcaneonavicular ligament

Inferior calcaneonavicular ligament

Also shares ligamentous support of subtalar joint & calcaneocuboid joint

TRANSVERSE TARSAL JOINT (MIDTARSAL JOINT)

- ▶ Compound joint formed by Talonavicular and calcaneocuboid joints

    'S' shaped joint line dividing the hind foot from midfoot & forefoot

    JOINT STRUCTURE:-

    Formation:

    Proximally by anterior calcaneus

    Distally by posterior cuboid

    Configuration:

    Reciprocally concave-convex across both dimension

- ▶ JOINT STABILITY
    - ✓ Capsule
    - ✓ Ligaments:
        1. Calcanecuboid ligament
        2. Dorsal CC ligament
        3. Plantar CC ligament
        4. Long plantar ligament
- ▶ Joint Function :

    Axis :

    Longitudinal & oblique axis producing supination/pronation

    Longitudinal axis: Nearly horizontal being slightly inclined upward, hence inversion/ eversion being predominate

    Oblique axis: Nearly parallels of TCN joint

    Hence DF/PF & abduction/adduction being predominate

TARSOMETATARSAL JOINT

- ▶ <u>Joint structure:</u>

Type: plane synovial joint

Formation:
- ✓ Posteriorly by the distal tarsal row
- ✓ Anteriorly by the bases of the metatarsal
- ✓ 1st joint: b/w the base of the 1st metatarsal and medial
- ✓ cuneiform
- ✓ 2nd joint: b/w 2nd metatarsal & with the mortise formed
- ✓ by the middle cuneiform & medial & lateral cuneiform
- ✓ 3rd joint :b/w 3rd metatarsal & lateral cuneiform
- ✓ 4th joint: b/w bases of the 4th and 5th metatarsal with
- ✓ cuboid

Ligaments:
- ✓ Dorsal ligament
- ✓ Plantar ligament
- ✓ Interosseous ligament
- ✓ Deep transverse ligament

▶ JOINT FUNCTION:

Axes:

Unique but not fully independent axis of motion

Ray:
- ✓ 1st ray :inclined so that in DF there is inversion & slight adduction
- ✓ 5th ray: inclined so that in DF there is eversion & slight abduction
- ✓ 3rd ray: axis coincides with the coronal axis so predominately there is DF and PF
- ✓ 4th ray: axis similar to but not as steep as 5th so that in DF there is slight eversion
- ✓ 2nd ray :axis inclined but not as oblique as 1st

Supination twist:

Inversion rotation around an hypothetical axis at 2nd ray

Weight Bearing ------→Hind Foot Pronation------→If Range not sufficient----→Medial side will press-→ Lateral side will left---→1st & 2nd Ray DF & 4th & 5th Ray PF------→Inversion-→In an attempt to maintain contact with ground.

Pronation twist:

Eversion accompanying the PF of the 1st & 2nd ray & DF of the 4th & 5th ray

METATARSOPHALANGEAL JOINT

- ▶ 5 metatarsophalangeal joint
- ▶ Type of joint:

Condyloid synovial joint

- ▶ Degree of freedom: 2 degrees of freedom DF/PF
  Abduction/Adduction
- ▶ Joint structure:

Formation :
- Proximally by head of metatarsal
- Distally by base of the phalanxes

Length of metatarsal:
- 2nd>1st>3rd>4th>5th: index minus foot
- 1st=2nd>3rd>4th>5th: index plus minus foot

1st>2nd>3rd>4th>5th: index plus foot

STABILITY:

plantar plate

plantar pad

collateral ligament

deep transverse metatarsal ligament

Plantar plate:

Fibrocartilaginous structure in 4 lesser toes

Connected

   Distally to base of proximal phalanx

   Proximally blend with the jt. capsule & with the interconnecting deep transverse ligament

Functions:
1. protects wt. bearing surface of the metatarsal head
2. provides stability to the MTP joints
3. helps to maintain the tendon position
4. helps in maintatning the small but dynamic BOS afforded by the toes

Metatarsal break :

Definition:

Single axis that lies through the 2nd -5th metatarsal heads & around which wt. bearing toe extension occurs

1. Range:
2. 54- 73 degrees compared to the long axis of the foot

Plantar aponeurosis:

Deep fascia covering the sole which is triangular in shape

Attachment:
- Proximally to the medial tubercle of the calcaneum,
- Distally Divides into 5 processes near the head of the metatarasal bones
- Each proceses splits into superficial and deep slips.
- Superficial slip is attached to the skin
- Deep slip divides into 2 parts which embrace the flexor tendons

MUSCLES OF THE ANKLE JOINT

Ankle plantar flexors:

   Principle muscles:
- Gastronemius
- Soleus

   Accessory muscles:
- Plantaris
- Tibialis posterior
- Flexor hallucis longus
- Flexor digitorum longus

▶ Ankle dorsiflexors:

   Principal muscles:
- Tibialis anterior

   Accessory muscles:
- Extensor hallucis longus
- Extensor digitorum longus
- Peroneus tertius

▶ Inversion:
- Tibialis anterior
- Tibialis posterior

- ✓ Flexor hallucis longus
- ✓ Flexor digitorum longus

Eversion :
- ✓ Peroneus longus
- ✓ Peroneus tertius

PATHOMECHANICS OF ANKLE AND FOOT

PES PLANUS: Abnormal pronation of the foot is called as pes planus

PES CAVUS: Abnormal highly arched foot is called as pes cavus.

FUNCTIONAL FOOT DISORDER:

VARUS: A varus position is an inverted position of the foot relative to the next

Rear foot varus: Inversion of the rearfoot relative to the to the ground.

Forefoot varus: Inverted position of the forefoot relative to the rearfoot at the level of midtarsal joint

Valgus: It is an everted position of one part relative to the next

Rearfoot valgus: Everted position of the foot relative to the leg

Forefoot valgus : Everted position of the forefoot relative to the rearfoot at the level of midtarsal joint

Compensated congenital gastronemius equinus: Due inadequate amount of ankle joint DF in developing child or adult

ROM of ankle joint <5 degrees with knee in extension & subtalar joint in the neutral position

ST jt. pronation which unlocks the midtarsal joint. allows independent DF of forefoot relative to the rear foot

CALCANEAL SPUR: Characterized by pain at the plantar medial aspect of calcaneus at the level of medial tubercle.

CLAWTOE DEFORMITY: Flexion at the proximal and distal interphalangeal joints of second through fifth digits

CUNEIFORM EXOSTOSIS: A bony prominence at the base of the first metatarsal at its articulation with the distal aspect of the 1st cuneiform is known as exostosis

HALLUX EXTENSUS: Dorsiflexed position of hallux (greater than 180 degrees) with an increased degree of hallux motion

HALLUX LIMITUS: Restriction of 1st MTP joint , less than the normal range of 65-75 degrees of dorsiflexion

HALLUX VALGUS: An apparent enlargement overlying the medial or dorso medial aspect of the 1st metatarsal leading outwrd bending og hallux

HAMMER TOE DEF ORMITY: Deformity of lesser toes, Flexion of PIP joint and hyperextension of MTP & DIP joints.

PLANTAR FASCITIS: Irritation of plantar fascia commonly involving the medial slip caused by the overstressing of the fascia.

PLANTAR TYLOMAS: Hyper keratotic lesions that develop secondary to abnormal shearing force over bony prominence

TAILOR'S BUNION: Painful enlargement or prominence of 5th metatarsal head

Refrences:

1. Nigg, B.M. and Herzog, W. (eds) (1999) *Biomechanics of the Musculoskeletal System*, Chichester: Wiley.
2. Frankel VH, Nordin M (eds): Basic *Biomechanics of the Skeletal System*. Philadelphia, PA, Lea & Febiger, 1980
3. P. Levangie , C. Norkin,2000, *Joint Structure and Function: A Comprehensive Analysis*, F.A. Davis Company.
4. Inman, V.T. (1976) *The Joints of the Ankle*, Baltimore, MD: Williams & Wilkins
5. Knudson, D.V. and Morrison, C.S. (2002) *Qualitative Analysis of Human Movement*, 2nd edn, Champaign, IL: Human Kinetics
6. DiStefano, V. (1981). Anatomy and biomechanics of the ankle and foot. *Athletic Training*, 16:43-47.
7. Czerniecki, J. M. (1988). Foot and ankle biomechanics in walking and running. *American Journal of Physical Medicine and Rehabilitation*, 67:246-25
8. Apkarian, J., et al. (1989). Three-dimensional kinematic and dynamic model of the lower limb. *Journal of Biomechanics*, 22:143-155.
9. Beynnon, B. D., et al. (2001). Ankle ligament injury risk factors: A prospective study of college athletes. *Journal of Orthopaedic Research*, 19:213-220.
10. Brown, L. P., Yavarsky, P. (1987). Locomotor biomechanics and pathomechanics: A review. *Journal of Orthopaedic and Sports Physical Therapy*, 9:3-10
11. Donatelli, R (1987). Abnormal biomechanics of the foot and ankle. *Journal of Orthopaedic and Sports Physical Therapy*, 9:11-15
12. Dave Thompson(2001) Retrieved from http://moon.ouhsc.edu/dthompso/namics/lecsked.htm

BIOMECHANICS OF TRUNK

SPINAL REGIONS

- HEAD (caput)
  The skull articulates with the top of the spine at the atlanto-occipital (AO) joint. Many muscles that cross the AO joint and move the head on the rest of the spine bear the word "capitis" in their names.
- CERVICAL: A curve that is ordinarily lordotic
- THORACIC: A curve that is ordinarily kyphotic
- LUMBAR: A curve that is ordinarily lordotic
- SACRAL: The five sacral segments are fused. However, motion occurs at the lumbosacral (L5-S1) and sacroiliac (SI) joints.

Axes of motion at intervertebral joints

JOINT	AXIS	MOTION
Atlanto-occipital(AO) lateral view	lateral	flexion/extension
	AP	lateral flexion (limited)
Atlanto-axial (AA)	vertical	rotation
Intervertebral joints below C2*	vertical	rotation
	AP	lateral flexion
	lateral	flexion/extension

*Below C2, all the intervertebral joints are functionally triaxial:

Vertical Axis	Located approximately through the posterior portion of the annulus fibrosis
Antero-Posterior (AP) axis	through center of vertebral disc
Lateral Axis	located approximately through the posterior portion of the annulus fibrosis

Pelvic motion requires motion at the surrounding joints

When a person stands, with both lower limbs fixed on a surface, pelvic motion requires hip motion. If the shoulders remain fixed as well, pelvic motion requires lumbar motion. These relationships occur in three planes.

SAGITTAL	lumbar flexion decreased lumbar lordosis posterior pelvic tilt hip extension	lumbar extension increased lumbar lordosis anterior pelvic tilt hip flexion

FRONTAL	if pelvis is low on left, high on right:
	    right intervertebral lateral flexion (sidebending)
	    right hip joint adduction
	    left hip joint abduction	

TRANSVERSE	left forward pelvic rotation =leftward lumbar rotation complementary hip rotation	

SACROILIAC (SI) JOINT

- Planar joint with complex contoured joint surface.
- Motions include:
    - sacral torsions
    - Innominate Rotations
        - ✓ Anterior Innominate rotation
        - ✓ Posterior Innominate rotation

Ligaments restrain intervertebral motion

- Anterior spinal ligaments (those located anterior to the spine's lateral or flexion-extension axis) elongate with and, therefore, limit extension:
    - ✓ Anterior longitudinal ligament
- Posterior spinal ligaments (those located posterior to the spine's lateral or flexion-extension axis) elongate with and, therefore, limit flexion:

✓ Posterior longitudinal lig. (2)
✓ Ligamentum flavum (3)
✓ Interspinous lig.(4)
✓ Supraspinous lig.(5)
✓ Ligamentum nuchae (an elaboration of the supraspinous ligament in the cervical region)
✓ Intertransverse lig.* (6)
✓ Facet (zygapophysial) joint capsules (7)

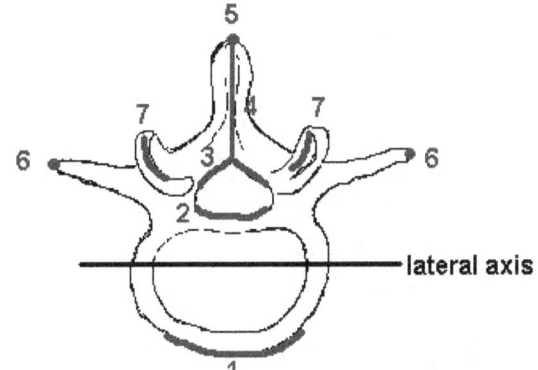

*Because of their lateral location, intertransverse ligaments (6) limit side bending to the opposite side, around the intervertebral joint's A-P axis.

Posterior ligamentous structures that are extrinsic to the spine also elongate with and prevent flexion:

- Thoracolumbar fascia

FORCES PRODUCE MOVEMENT IN THE SPINE

Forces can be gravitational or muscular

1. In sagittal plane (around lateral axis)
    - Anterior forces cause flexion
    - Posterior forces cause extension
2. In frontal plane (around a-p axis)
    - Forces to left of axis cause left sidebending.
    - Forces to right of axis cause right sidebending.
3. In transverse plane (around vertical / longitudinal axis)
    - Any force that is not parallel to the spine will cause rotation.

BIOMECHANICS OF RESPIRATION

1. The bottom line
    - ✓ Matter flows from areas of high pressure to areas of low pressure.
    - ✓ When the intrathoracic pressure is low, air (at atmospheric pressure) flows into the lung.
    - ✓ When the intrathoracic pressure is high, air (at atmospheric pressure) flows out of the lung.

2. Intrathoracic volume and pressure

    The Ideal Gas Law:

    $PV = nRT$

    $PV/nT = R$

    (where R is the 'gas constant')

    Implications:
    - At a given temperature, [pressure x volume] is a constant quantity
    - Pressure and volume vary inversely. An increase in one is associated with a decrease in the other.

3. THORACIC ANATOMY

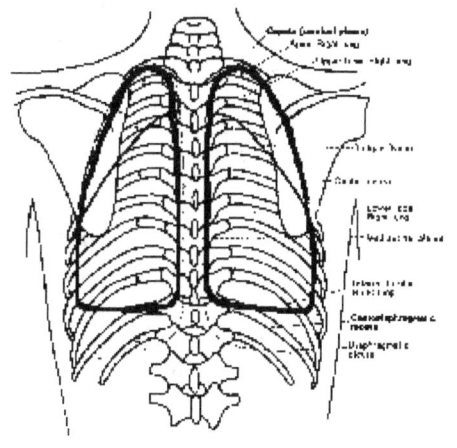

The T10 spinous process is a posterior surface landmark for the inferior boundary of lung substance.

- base of scapular spine is at T4
- inferior angle of scapula is at T8

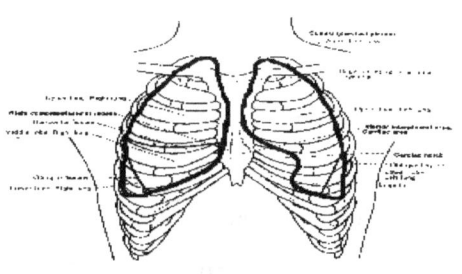

The xiphoid process is an anterior surface landmark for the inferior boundary of lung substance.

4. Thoracic movement during inspiration and expiration

INSPIRATION	EXPIRATION
DIAPHRAGM DESCENDS	DIAPHRAGM ASCENDS
RIBCAGE ELEVATES AND/OR EXPANDS	RIBCAGE DESCENDS AND/OR CONTRACTS
INCREASED INTRATHORACIC VOLUME	DECREASED INTRATHORACIC VOLUME
DECREASED INTRATHORACIC PRESSURE	INCREASED INTRATHORACIC PRESSURE
'HIGH PRESSURE' EXTERIOR AIR FLOWS INTO 'LOW PRESSURE' LUNG.	'HIGH PRESSURE' AIR IN LUNG FLOWS OUT TOWARD 'LOW PRESSURE' EXTERIOR.

5. Muscles of respiration

	Inspiration	Expiration
Quiet (primary muscles)	diaphragm external intercostals	elastic recoil of lung tissue surface tension gravity on ribs internal intercostals

Forced (secondary or accessory muscles)	sternocleidomastoideus
	scalenes
	pectoralis major
	pectoralis minor
	serratus anterior
	serratus posterior superior
	upper iliocostalis
		abdominals
		   external oblique
		   internal oblique
		   rectus abdominus
		lower iliocostalis
		lower longissimus
		serratus posterior inferior

6. THE DIAPHRAGM

Shortening of diaphragmatic fibers pulls

1. Inferiorly on central tendon
2. Superiorly on lower ribs

During inspiration, the diaphragm's central tendon descends until it is fixed or stabilized by forces that develop in:

1. Elongated mediastinal structures, which pull upward on the diaphragm
2. Compressed abdominal contents, which push upward on the descending diaphragm

When the central tendon becomes stable, it is still superior to the diaphragm's mobile attachments on the lower ribs. Therefore, the diaphragm's muscular lines of application elevate the lower ribs. Because of the orientation of the lower ribs' attachments to the vertebrae, rib elevation expands the thorax' lateral dimensions.

Refrences:

1. Nigg, B.M. and Herzog, W. (eds) (1999) *Biomechanics of the Musculoskeletal System*, Chichester: Wiley.
2. Frankel VH, Nordin M (eds): *Basic Biomechanics of the Skeletal System*.Philadelphia, PA, Lea & Febiger, 1980
3. P. Levangie, C. Norkin,2000, *Joint Structure and Function: A Comprehensive Analysis*, F.A. Davis Company.
4. Knudson, D.V. and Morrison, C.S. (2002) *Qualitative Analysis of Human Movement*, 2nd edn, Champaign, IL: Human Kinetics.
5. Blaber, M. (1996). The ideal gas equation. Retrieved from October 31, 2001 from Florida State University, General Chemistry 1, A Virtual Textbook Web site: http://wine1.sb.fsu.edu/chm1045/notes/Gases/IdealGas/Gases04.htm
6. Clemente, C.D. (1981). Anatomy. (2nd ed.). Baltimore: Urban and Schwarzenberg.
7. Kapandji, I.A. (1974). Functional components of the vertebral column. In I.A. Kapandji, *The physiology of the joints: Vol. 3*. The trunk and the vertebral column. New York: Churchill Livingstone.
8. Poole, D.C., Sexton, W.L., Farkas, G.A., Powers, S.K., Reid, M.B. (1997). Diaphragm structure and function in health and disease. *Medicine and Science in Sports and Exercise*, 29, 738-54. (full text version is available on Medline; Unique Identifier: 97362737).
9. Dave Thompson(2001) Retrieved from http://moon.ouhsc.edu/dthompso/namics/lecsked.htm
10. Rasch, P.J., & Burke, R.K. (1978). *Kinesiology and applied anatomy (6th ed.)*. Philadelphia: Lea and Febiger.

GAIT

Normal Gait
- Series of rhythmical, alternating movements of the trunk & limbs which result in the forward progression of the center of gravity

Gait Cycle
- Single sequence of functions by **one limb**
- Begins when reference font contacts the ground
- Ends with subsequent floor contact of the same foot

Step Length
- Distance between corresponding successive **points of heel contact of the opposite feet**
- Rt step length = Lt step length (in normal gait)

Stride Length
Distance between successive points of heel contact of the **same foot**
- Double the step length (in normal gait)

Walking Base
- Side-to-side distance between the line of the two feet
- Also known as 'stride width'

Cadence
- Number of steps per unit time
- Normal: 100 – 115 **steps/min**
- Cultural/social variations

Comfortable Walking Speed (CWS)
- Least energy consumption per unit distance
- Average = **80 m/min** (~ 5 km/h, ~ 3 mph)

Phases:

- **Stance Phase:**   **Swing Phase:**
  reference limb   reference limb
  in contact   not in contact
  with the floor   with the floor

Support:
(1) <u>Single Support</u>: Only one foot in contact with the floor

(2) <u>Double Support</u>: Both feet in contact with floor

A. <u>Stance phase:</u>

1. **Heel contact**: 'Initial contact'
2. **Foot-flat**: 'Loading response', initial contact of forefoot w. ground
3. **Midstance**: Greater trochanter in alignment vertical bisector of foot
4. **Heel-off**: 'Terminal stance'
5. **Toe-off**: 'Pre-swing'

B. <u>Swing phase:</u>

1. **Acceleration**: 'Initial swing'
2. **Midswing**: swinging limb overtakes the limb in stance
3. **Deceleration**: 'Terminal swing'

Time Frame:

A. Stance vs. Swing:
- Stance phase = 60% of gait cycle
- Swing phase = 40%

B. Single vs. Double support:
- Single support = 40% of gait cycle
- Double support = 20%

With increasing walking speeds:
- Stance phase: decreases
- Swing phase: increases
- Double support: decreases

Running:
- By definition: walking without double support
- Ratio stance/swing reverses
- Double support disappears. 'Double swing' develops

With increasing walking speeds:
- Stance phase: decreases
- Swing phase: increases
- Double support: decreases

Path of Center of Gravity

Center of Gravity (CG):

- ✓ midway between the hips
- ✓ Few cm in front of S2
▶ Least energy consumption if CG travels in straight line

A. <u>Vertical displacement</u>:
- ✓ Rhythmic up & down movement
- ✓ Highest point: midstance
- ✓ Lowest point: double support
- ✓ Average displacement: 5cm
- ✓ Path: extremely smooth sinusoidal curve

B. <u>Lateral displacement</u>:
- ✓ Rhythmic side-to-side movement
- ✓ Lateral limit: midstance
- ✓ Average displacement: 5cm
- ✓ Path: extremely smooth sinusoidal curve

Determinants of Gait :
- ✓ Six optimizations used to minimize excursion of CG in vertical & horizontal planes
- ✓ Reduce significantly energy consumption of ambulation

  (1) <u>Pelvic rotation</u>:
  - ○ Forward rotation of the pelvis in the horizontal plane approx. 8° on the swing-phase side
  - ✓ Reduces the angle of hip flexion & extension
  - ✓ Enables a slightly longer step-length w/o further lowering of CG

  (2) <u>Pelvic tilt</u>:
  - ✓ 5° dip of the swinging side (i.e. hip adduction)
  - ✓ In standing, this dip is a positive Trendelenberg sign
  - ✓ Reduces the height of the apex of the curve of CG

  (3) <u>Knee flexion in stance phase</u>:
  - ✓ Approx. 20° dip
  - ✓ Shortens the leg in the middle of stance phase
  - ✓ Reduces the height of the apex of the curve of CG

  (4) <u>Ankle mechanism</u>:
  - ✓ Lengthens the leg at heel contact

- ✓ Smoothens the curve of CG
- ✓ Reduces the lowering of CG

(5) <u>Foot mechanism</u>:
- ✓ Lengthens the leg at toe-off as ankle moves from dorsiflexion to plantarflexion
- ✓ Smoothens the curve of CG
- ✓ Reduces the lowering of CG

(6) <u>Lateral displacement of body</u>:
- ✓ The normally narrow width of the walking base minimizes the lateral displacement of CG
- ✓ Reduced muscular energy consumption due to reduced lateral acceleration & deceleration

COMMON GAIT ABNORMALITIES:

A. Antalgic Gait
- ✓ Gait pattern in which stance phase on affected side is shortened
- ✓ Corresponding increase in stance on unaffected side

B. Lateral Trunk bending
- ✓ Trendelenberg gait
- ✓ Usually unilateral
- ✓ Bilateral = waddling gait
- ✓ Common causes:
    - A. Painful hip
    - B. Hip abductor weakness
    - C. Leg-length discrepancy
    - D. Abnormal hip joint

C. Functional Leg-Length Discrepancy
- ✓ Swing leg: longer than stance leg
- ✓ 4 common compensations:
    - A. Circumduction
    - B. Hip hiking
    - C. Steppage
    - D. Vaulting

D. Increased Walking Base

- ✓ Normal walking base: 5-10 cm
- ✓ Common causes:
  - Deformities   Abducted hip and valgus knee
  - Instability
    - ▶ Cerebellar ataxia
    - ▶ Proprioception deficits

E. Inadequate Dorsiflexion Control

- ✓ In stance phase (Heel contact – Foot flat):
  - **Foot slap**
- ✓ In swing phase (mid-swing):
  - **Toe drag**
- ✓ Causes:
  - Weak Tibialis Ant.
  - Spastic plantarflexors

F. Excessive knee extension

- ✓ Loss of normal knee flexion during stance phase
- ✓ Knee may go into hyperextension
- ✓ Genu recurvatum: hyperextension deformity of knee
- ✓ Common causes:
  - Quadriceps weakness (mid-stance)
  - Quadriceps spasticity (mid-stance)
  - Knee flexor weakness (end-stance)

References:

1. Nigg, B.M. and Herzog, W. (eds) (1999) *Biomechanics of the Musculoskeletal System*, Chichester: Wiley.
2. Frankel VH, Nordin M (eds): *Basic Biomechanics of the Skeletal System.* Philadelphia, PA, Lea & Febiger, 1980
3. P. Levangie, C. Norkin, 2000, *Joint Structure and Function: A Comprehensive Analysis*, F.A. Davis Company.
4. Knudson, D.V. and Morrison, C.S. (2002) *Qualitative Analysis of Human Movement*, 2nd edn, Champaign, IL: Human Kinetics
5. Dave Thompson(2001) Retrieved from http://moon.ouhsc.edu/dthompso/namics/lecsked.htm

POSTURE

Posture is a position or attitude of the body, the relative arrangement of body parts for a specific activity, or a characteristic manner of bearing one's body.

Types of Posture

STATIC POSTURE:-

In static postures the body and its segments are aligned and maintained in certain positions.

E.g. Standing, Kneeling, Lying and Sitting.

DYNAMIC POSTURE:-

It refers to postures in which the body or its segments are moving.

E.g. Walking, Running, Jumping, Throwing and Lifting.

For a good posture, the following are very much important:-

Base Of Support (BOS): The human species' BOS, defined by an area bounded posteriorly by the tips of the heels and anteriorly by a line joining the tips of the toes, is considerably smaller than the quadrupedal base.

Centre Of Gravity (COG): The human's COG, which is sometimes referred to as the body's Center Of Mass (COM), is located within the body approximately at the level of the second sacral segment, a location that is relatively distant from the BOS.

- Despite the instability caused by a small BOS and a high COG, maintaining stability in the erect posture requires very little energy expenditure in the form of muscle contraction.
- Can be either static or dynamic, and refers to a person's ability to maintain stability of the body and body segments in response to forces that threaten to disturb the body's structural equilibrium.
- The CNS interprets and organizes inputs from the various structures and systems and selects responses based on past experience and the goal of the response.
    - Reactive (Compensatory) Responses occur as reactions to external forces that displace the body's COG.
    - Proactive (Anticipatory) Responses occur in anticipation of internally generated destabilizing forces such as raising one's arms to catch a ball or bending forward to tie one's shoes.

Major Goals and Basic Elements of Control

Major goals of postural control in the erect position are:
- To control the body's orientation in space,
- Maintain the body's COG over the BOS, and
- Stabilize the head with respect to the vertical so that the eye gaze is approximately oriented.
- According to DiFabio, stabilizing the head with respect to the vertical is the primary goal of postural regulation.

- Maintenance and control of posture depends on the integrity of the CNS, visual system, vestibular system, and the musculoskeletal system.
- Major Goals and Basic Elements of Control
- In addition, postural control depends on information from receptors located in and around the joints (in joint capsules, tendons, and ligaments) as well as on the soles of the feet.
- The CNS must be able to detect and predict instability and must be able to respond to all of this input with appropriate output to maintain the equilibrium of the body.
- Muscle Synergies
- A normally functioning CNS selects the appropriate combination of muscles to complete the task based on an analysis of sensory inputs.
- Perturbation: It is any sudden change in conditions that displaces the body posture away from equilibrium.
    - Sensory Perturbation:- It might be caused by altering of visual input such as might occur when one's eyes are covered unexpectedly.
    - Mechanical Perturbation:- These are displacements that involve direct changes in the relationship of COG to the Base of Support (BOS). These displacements are caused either by movements of body segments or of the entire body.
- The postural responses to perturbation caused by either platform movement or by pushes and pulls are reactive or compensatory responses in that they are Involuntary Reactions. These postural responses are referred to in the literature as either Synergies or Strategies.
- Fixed-Support Synergies:-
    - These are patterns of muscle activity in which the BOS remains fixed during the perturbation and recovery of equilibrium.
    - E.g. Ankle Synergy and Hip Synergy.

Ankle Synergy consists of discrete bursts of muscle activity on either the anterior or posterior aspects of the body that occur in a distal-to-proximal pattern in response to forward and backward movements of the surrounding platform, respectively.

Hip Synergy consists of discrete bursts of muscle activity on the side of the body opposite to the ankle pattern in a proximal-to-distal pattern of activation.

Change-in-Support Strategies:-

- The change-in-support strategies include Stepping (forward, backward or sidewise) and Grasping (using one's hands to grab a bar or other fixed support) in response to movements of the platform.
- Change-in-support synergies are the only synergies that are successful in maintaining stability in the instance of a large perturbation.

Head Stabilizing Strategies:-

- These strategies occur in anticipation of the initiation of internally generated forces.
- These are used to maintain the head during sustained movement of the body, such as walking, whereas the previously described strategies are used to maintain the body in a static equilibrium situation.
- The Head Stabilization in Space (HSS) strategy is a modification of head position in anticipation of displacements of the body's COG. The anticipatory adjustments to head position are independent of trunk motion.
- The Head Stabilization on Trunk (HST) strategy is one in which the head and trunk move as a single unit.

Kinetics and Kinematics of Posture

The external forces considered here are Inertia, Gravity and Ground Reaction Forces (GRFs).

- Generally, inertial forces are ignored in static postures because little or no acceleration is occurring except during postural sway. In the erect standing posture the body undergoes a constant swaying motion called Postural Sway or Sway Envelope.
- Whenever the body contacts the ground, the ground pushes back on the body. This force is known as the Ground Reaction Force or GRF.

The **composite** or **resultant ground reaction force vector (GRVF)** is equal in magnitude but opposite in direction to the gravitational force in the erect static standing posture.

The point of application of the GRFV is at the body's Center of Gravity (COP), which is located in the foot in unilateral stance and between the feet in bilateral standing postures.

Optimal or Ideal Posture

- An Ideal Posture is one in which the body segments are aligned vertically and the LOG passes through all joint axes.
- In the normal optimal standing posture the gravitational torques are small and can be balanced by counter-torques generated by passing ligamentous tension, passive muscle tension, and a minimal amount of muscle activity. The body segments in the normal optimal posture are in or near vertical alignment.
- If faulty postures are habitual and assumed continually on a daily basis, the body will not recognize these faulty postures as abnormal and over time structural adaptations will occur.

Analysis of Posture

Posture analysis can be done in any ways, some of which are described below:-

1. Plumb Line
2. Grid Method
3. Radiographic Techniques
4. Visual Analysis
5. Set of Six Blocks
6. Peg Stand

Refrences:

1. Nigg, B.M. and Herzog, W. (eds) (1999) *Biomechanics of the Musculoskeletal System*, Chichester: Wiley.
2. Dave Thompson(2001) Retrieved from http://moon.ouhsc.edu/dthompso/namics/lecsked.htm

3. Frankel VH, Nordin M (eds): Basic *Biomechanics of the Skeletal System*.Philadelphia, PA, Lea & Febiger, 1980
4. P. Levangie , C. Norkin,2000, *Joint Structure and Function: A Comprehensive Analysis*, F.A. Davis Company.
5. Knudson, D.V. and Morrison, C.S. (2002) *Qualitative Analysis of Human Movement*, 2nd edn, Champaign, IL: Human Kinetics

BIOMECHANICS OF PROSTHETIC

Prosthetic alignment alters gait by manipulating the position of LE and prosthetic joints with respect to ground reaction forces (GRF).

In normal gait, from initial contact through loading response,

- Ground reaction (GRF) originates at the heel, passing posteriorly to the ankle and knee joints.
- This produces knee flexion and ankle plantar flexion, which are controlled respectively by the knee extensors and ankle dorsiflexors.

From midstance though preswing,

- The GRF moves anterior to the ankle, producing ankle DF that must be controlled by the plantar flexors.
- The ankle gradually dorsiflexes (under eccentric PF control), then plantar flexes (owing to concentric PF activity).
- Forward tibial inclination permits the heel to rise and the GRF to fall behind the knee, inducing preswing knee flexion.

In gait with a prosthetic foot,

- The shape and density of the prosthetic heel (e.g. cushion on a SACH foot or PF bumper on a single-axis foot) allows the front of the foot to settle on the floor during loading response (in "pseudoplantar flexion").
- A relatively rigid prosthetic ankle or DF bumper controls movement of GRF over foot through midstance.
- Length of keel structure determines timing of heel rise.
- The location of the trochanter-knee-ankle (TKA) line determines "tradeoff" during stance between:
    - inherent knee stability and
    - voluntary control of prosthetic knee.

The way a prosthesis behaves during gait depends on the relative length of what prosthetists call the heel and toe levers.

- "Heel lever": roughly the perpendicular distance from heel cushion to center of socket.
- "Toe lever": roughly the perpendicular distance from center of socket to end of keel.

Changes in these levers produce predictable changes in an amputee's gait pattern:

SHORTENING the heel lever:
1. Locates the GRF more anteriorly with respect to the knee during loading response and midstance, thus producing knee extension earlier in the gait cycle.
2. Increases the toe lever, which sustains knee extension later in the gait cycle. If the toe lever is too long, the individual may be unable to initiate pre swing knee flexion.

LENGTHENING the heel lever:
1. Locates the GRF more posteriorly with respect to the knee at initial contact (heel strike), thus producing a larger knee flexion moment during loading response.
2. Decreases the toe lever, which causes the knee to flex earlier in midstance or terminal stance. "Drop off" results if the toe lever is too short and the knee flexes before the person is ready to accept weight on the opposite leg.

The prosthetist can alter heel and toe levers in predictable ways by changing the relationship between the socket and foot.

- To decrease heel lever:
- To increase heel lever:

Socket and foot alignment also influence forces and pressures that the socket places on the residual limb.

References

1. Cerny, K, et al. (1990). Effect of an unrestricted knee-ankle-foot orthosis on the stance phase gait in healthy persons. Orthopedics, 13:1121-1127.
2. Clark, T E., et al. (1983). The effects of shoe design parameters on rearfoot control in running. Medicine and Science in Sports and Exercise, 5:376-381
3. Czerniecki, J. M. (1988). Foot and ankle biomechanics in walking and running. American Journal of Physical Medicine and Rehabilitation, 67:246-252.
4. Collins, N., Bisset, L., McPoil, T. and Vicenzino, B. (2007) 'Foot orthoses in lower limb overuse conditions: a systematic review and meta-analysis', *Foot and Ankle International*, 28: 396–412.
5. Tiberio,D. 1988.Pathomechanical structure of foot deformities,Physical Therapy,68,1840-9
6. Dave Thompson(2001) Retrieved from http://moon.ouhsc.edu/dthompso/namics/lecsked.htm